MEDICAL PARASITOLOGY

Ralph Muller BSc, PhD, FIBiol, CBiol
Director, CAB International Institute of Parasitology
St Albans, UK

John R Baker BSc, PhD, DSc, MA, FIBiol
Former Reader in Parasitic Protozoology
University of London, UK

J.B. Lippincott Company   PHILADELPHIA

Gower Medical Publishing   LONDON • NEW YORK

Distributed in USA and Canada by:
J. B. Lippincott Company
East Washington Square
Philadelphia, PA 19105
USA

Distributed in UK and Continental Europe by:
Harper & Row Ltd
Middlesex House
34-42 Cleveland Street
London W1P 5FB, UK

Distributed in Australia and New Zealand by:
Harper & Row (Australasia) Pty Ltd
PO Box 226
Artarmon, NSW 2064
Australia

Distributed in Southeast Asia, Hong Kong, India and Pakistan by:
Harper & Row Publishers (Asia) Pte Ltd
37 Jalan Pemimpin 02-01
Singapore 2057

Distributed in Japan by:
Igaku Shoin Ltd
Tokyo International
PO Box 5063
Tokyo
Japan

Distributed in Philippines/Guam, Middle East, Latin America and Africa by:
Harper & Row International
10 East 53rd Street
New York, NY. 10022
USA

Library of Congress Catalog Number: 88–81420

British Library Cataloguing in Publication Data
    Muller, Ralph
    Medical parasitology.
    1. Man. Parasitic diseases
    I. Title II. Baker, John R. (John Robin), 1931-
    616.9'6

ISBN 0–397–44609–8

Printed in Hong Kong by Imago Publishing Ltd.
Originated in Hong Kong by Bright Arts (HK) Ltd.
Set in Bembo and News Gothic by M to N
Typesetters, London.

PROJECT TEAM
Publisher: Fiona Foley
Project Editors: Gillian Lancaster
                Marion Jowett
Design & Illustration: Ian Spick
Linework: Marion Tasker
        Mark Willey
        Jenni Miller
Production: Seamus Murphy
Index: Anita Reid

PREFACE

This book is intended primarily as an introductory text for undergraduate medical students. Parasitology has always been an important part of the curriculum in developing countries but, with the increase in air travel and the recent appearance of new opportunistic parasitic infections of man, a knowledge of parasites is needed by students in developed countries also. The book aims to provide a suitable depth of treatment for both postgraduate students taking courses which include parasitology, for example microbiology, tropical public health, or tropical medicine, and for undergraduate science students who study human parasitic diseases, perhaps as part of Third World studies.

The text is accompanied by numerous colour plates, which have been carefully chosen to reinforce the learning process, to help in the practical identification of the causative organisms, and to illustrate the damage they can do; clear and accurate diagrams of life cycles and distribution maps are also included. Care has been taken that all diagrams reflect current knowledge of the subject. We have included a comprehensive and up-to-date further reading list for those who wish to obtain more information on any aspect of the subject.

New techniques in molecular biology, such as infra-specific variation, immunodiagnosis, understanding of immune processes, and the prospects for vaccine production, are revolutionizing certain aspects of parasitology, and these are summarized in a final section.

Parasites and their vectors are considered in systematic order rather than under organs attacked since we consider this most appropriate for a non-clinical textbook. However, parasites, and the most important pathological effects they cause, are listed under the various organs and tissues of the body in a set of appendices.

While this book is intended as an introduction to the subject, we have attempted to incorporate some of our practical knowledge, since we both have extensive experience working in many countries of the developing world as research and field workers, as university teachers and as external examiners and have also acted as consultants to international agencies in the fight against parasitic diseases.

Ralph Muller
John R. Baker

ACKNOWLEDGEMENTS

It is a pleasure to thank colleagues for their criticisms of portions of this book, and in particular Dr R. P. Lane for his very valuable comments on the arthropods chapter. We have attempted to acknowledge the original source of all colour photographs other than those from our own collections and apologise if any attributions have been omitted.

Ralph Muller
John R. Baker

CONTENTS

1. PROTOZOA

INTRODUCTION

Protozoa are usually defined as single-celled animals, though some people prefer to regard them as non-cellular, that is, animals which have not become subdivided into cells. Both views are valid: structurally, protozoa resemble single metazoan cells, while functionally each is equivalent to a whole metazoan animal. The protozoan cell has a full complement of cellular organelles; nucleus, mitochondria, endoplasmic reticulum and Golgi apparatus (Fig. 1.1) together with specialized organelles in some groups, such as rhoptries, micronemes and the apical complex (Fig. 1.2).

There is no basic difference between protozoa and single-celled algae, although the latter can generally be distinguished by the possession of chloroplasts containing the green photosynthetic pigment chlorophyll. There are many unicellular organisms which are borderline; for example, within the genus *Euglena* there are both green and colourless species. Purists unite the single-celled animals and single-celled plants into one kingdom, the Protista. This is a valid view but for many practical purposes it is convenient to keep the protozoa separate, while always bearing in mind that the division is artificial. Trying to erect convenient boundaries in what is naturally a continuum is always likely to give rise to borderline cases, and demarcation disputes occur between phycologists and protozoologists, with each group laying claim to a particular organism. All the symbiotic protozoa are clearly animal-like in nature, none being photosynthetic and all depending on other organisms to provide them with ready-made foodstuffs — proteins, fats and carbohydrates — rather than building these up for themselves from simple compounds. The processes of digestion and respiration which protozoa use do not differ fundamentally from those adopted by metazoan cells; for

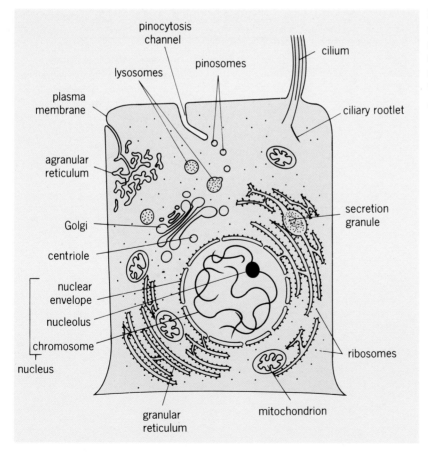

Fig. 1.1 Diagram of an idealized metazoan cell, showing intracellular organelles. Protozoa may contain some or all of these organelles, plus others not shown. (Modified from Vickerman & Cox, *The Protozoa*, John Murray, London, 1967.)

details of these processes, and of protozoan anatomy, the reader should consult the books suggested as further reading.

All protozoa, whether symbiotic or free-living, reproduce by some form of asexual division. Some also undergo a form of sexual reproduction, usually involving a division process after an exchange of genetic material mediated by the permanent or temporary fusion of two individuals of different sex or mating type.

Discussion of the detailed classification of the protozoa can be found in books recommended for further reading. It is sufficient here to note that protozoa can be broadly divided into five large groups, generally accorded the rank of phyla:

● Sarcomastigophora; forms whose main method of locomotion is by means of temporary extensions of the cell, known as pseudopodia (for example,

Entamoeba), or by the beating of long whip-like structures called flagella (for example, *Giardia*, *Trypanosoma*), or both.

● Apicomplexa; united by having in some stages of the life cycle a complex set of organelles, the apical complex, visible only by electron microscopy, at the anterior pole of the cell. All are symbiotic (for example, *Plasmodium*, *Toxoplasma*).

● Ciliophora; a very specialized group of highly sophisticated single-celled organisms whose common feature is the possession of large numbers of short hair-like extensions of the cell, cilia, the co-ordinated beating of which enables them to swim (for example, *Balantidium*).

● Two other groups entirely composed of highly specialized symbionts, the Microsporida and Myxozoa.

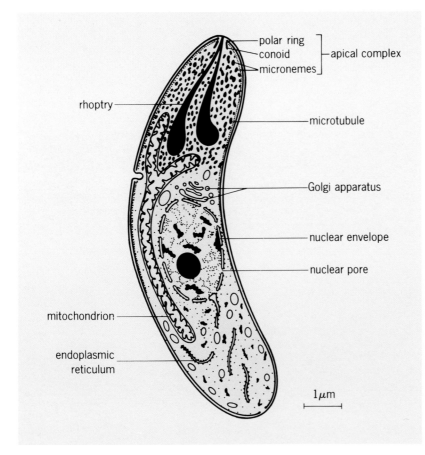

Fig. 1.2 Diagram of the merozoite form of a member of the phylum Apicomplexa. The micronemes and rhoptries are unique to the apicomplexans, and are concerned with penetration of host cells.

The only symbiotic protozoa important in human parasitology are those at least potentially harmful (pathogenic) to their hosts. There are other symbiotic protozoa, mostly living in the human gastrointestinal tract, that are harmless commensals and need to be differentiated from the potential pathogens when making a diagnosis. The true parasites are not necessarily always harmful to their hosts, for example *Entamoeba histolytica* (see page 47).

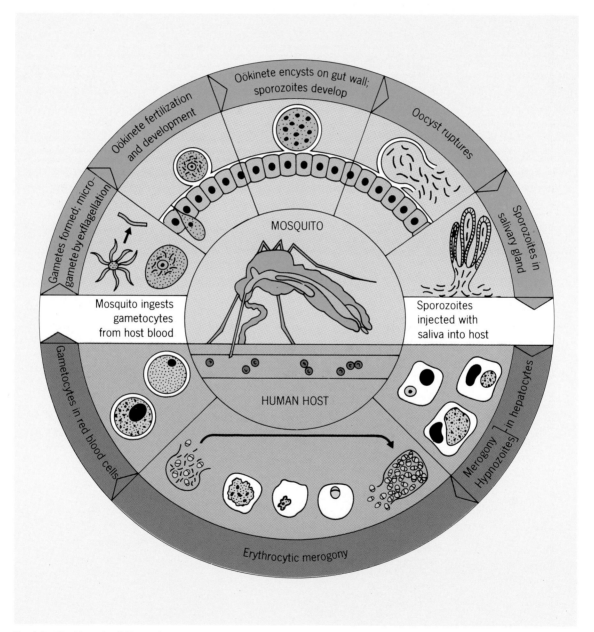

Fig. 1.3   The life cycle of *Plasmodium vivax*.

Symbiotic protozoa may be either obligate or facultative symbionts; all the forms discussed below are obligate symbionts for at least part of the life cycle.

PLASMODIUM

Causative organism	Disease
Plasmodium falciparum	Malignant tertian malaria
Plasmodium malariae	Quartan malaria
Plasmodium ovale	Ovale tertian malaria
Plasmodium vivax	Benign tertian malaria

Malaria is a disease which has been known for millennia: on some Egyptian papyri of around 1500 BC there are recognizable descriptions; Hippocrates, in about 400 BC, gave an accurate description of the disease. It was not until 1880, however, that the causative organisms were first seen and described by the French military doctor Alphonse Laveran (working in Algeria). Although Laveran suggested that mosquitoes might transmit the infection, another seventeen years were to elapse before this was first demonstrated, by Ronald Ross using malaria of birds. In 1898 the Italian group led by Battista Grassi

transmitted human malaria to a volunteer, and the life cycle in the vector insect and in human erythrocytes was elucidated. The 'missing stage' between infective mosquito bite and appearance of parasites in blood cells, the existence of which was proposed by Grassi, was not discovered (in human malaria) until 1948, when it was described by Henry Shortt and Cyril Garnham from a liver biopsy removed from a heroic volunteer.

Transmission and epidemiology

The life cycle of *Plasmodium vivax* is summarized in Fig. 1.3. The sexual stages (gametocytes) in human red blood cells develop further only if ingested by a female mosquito (male mosquitoes do not feed on blood) of the genus *Anopheles*. All the stages occurring in the human host are haploid, as are the male and female (or micro- and macro-) gametes formed in the mosquito's gut. The microgametes are formed by the exflagellation process and measure $20-25\mu m$ long (Fig. 1.4). When the gametes fuse, the resulting zygote is diploid, as is the motile ookinete (c.20 × $3\mu m$) into which it transforms (Fig. 1.5). The ookinete penetrates one of the cells forming the wall of the mosquito's stomach and encysts just beneath

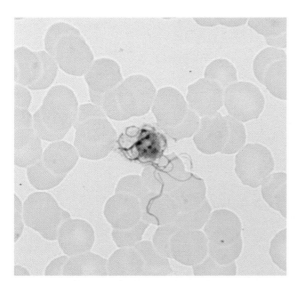

Fig. 1.4 Exflagellation; *P. vivax* microgametocyte producing eight long threadlike microgametes.

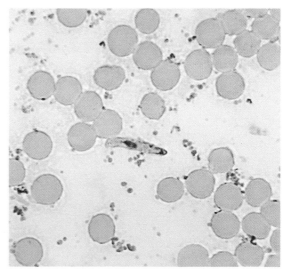

Fig. 1.5 Ookinete of *P. vivax*.

the basement membrane on the outer surface of the wall (Fig. 1.6). Fully grown oocysts measure up to 50μm in diameter. Each then begins a series of nuclear divisions, the first of which is a reduction (meiotic) division, followed by cytoplasmic cleavage to produce thousands of sporozoites, the process being known as sporogony; each sporozoite is, therefore, haploid and measures c.15μm long. Some of the sporozoites enter the lumen of the mosquito's salivary glands (Fig. 1.7) and are injected with the saliva when the insect next bites a mammal.

When sporozoites are injected into a susceptible species (man, or for *P. malariae*, the chimpanzee also) they rapidly (within 30 minutes) enter liver parenchyma cells. Whether they do this directly or via the phagocytic Kupffer cells which line the liver blood sinusoids is uncertain. They then (unless hypnozoites, see below) begin a process of multiple divisions known as merogony (or schizogony; Fig. 1.8). At this stage they are known as meronts ($50–60\mu$m in diameter when mature).

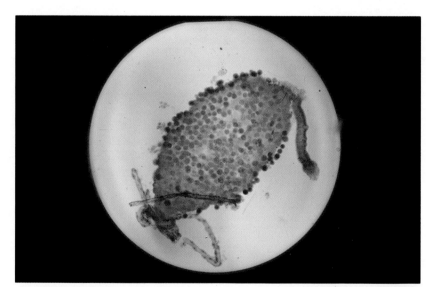
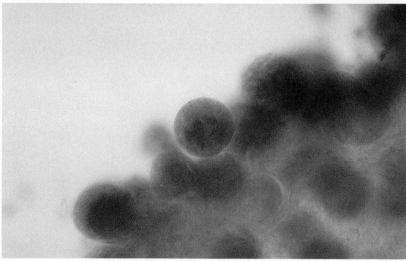

Fig. 1.6 Oocysts on the exterior surface of the mosquito midgut (upper), shown in more detail in the enlargement (lower).

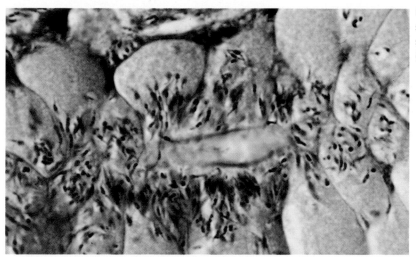

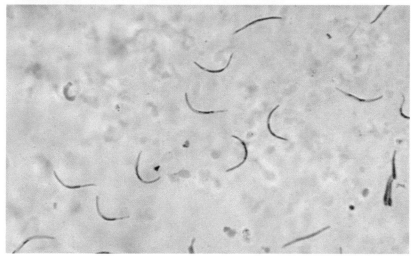

Fig. 1.7 Sporozoites in *Anopheles* salivary gland (upper) and in a smear from an infected gland (lower).

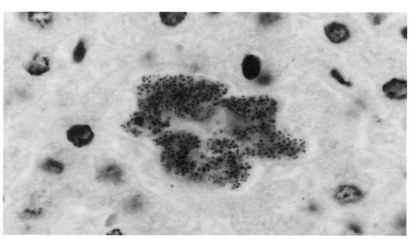

Fig. 1.8 Merogony. Section through an exoerythrocytic meront of *P. falciparum* in a hepatocyte from a human volunteer.

Merogony in liver cells results in the production of thousands of merozoites per meront. These merozoites penetrate red blood cells to become ring-form trophozoites, and thus enter the general circulation. They then undergo another phase of merogony, more limited in extent than that in the liver cells. As the parasites within the erythrocytes grow, they ingest and digest the host cell's haemoglobin; the indigestible iron-containing part of the haemoglobin molecule forms the characteristic brown or black malarial pigment.

The ring forms of *P. falciparum* (Fig. 1.9) are very small (1 μm in diameter), with a very thin circle of cytoplasm; some appear to have two nuclei, and some are closely pressed to the periphery of the cell (accolé forms). Meronts of *P. falciparum* are rarely seen in peripheral blood, because infected cells adhere to the endothelium of capillaries in the internal organs.

Ring forms of *P. vivax* (Fig. 1.10) are larger (2 μm in diameter), and as the parasite grows the infected cell becomes enlarged and develops red-staining Schüffner's dots on its surface; the growing parasite (trophozoite) is actively motile (hence the specific name) and thus often appears irregular in shape. The meronts are larger than those of *P. falciparum*.

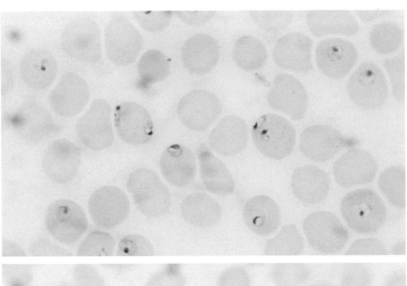
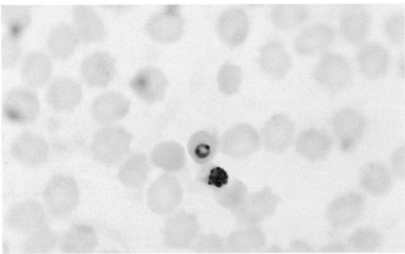

Fig. 1.9 *P. falciparum*: (upper) ring forms; (lower) an older ring form and a meront.

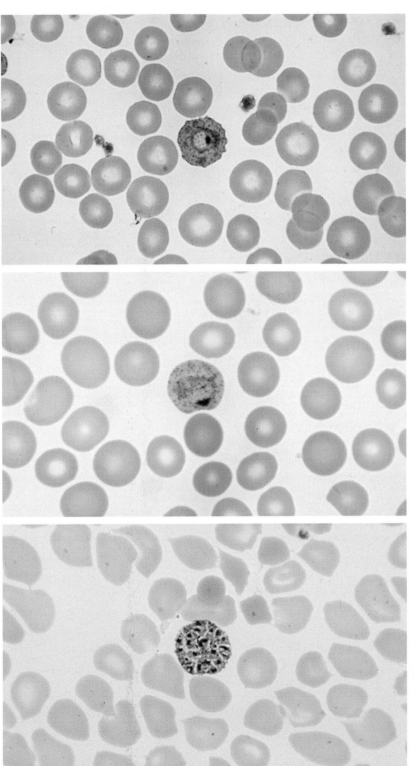

Fig. 1.10 *P. vivax*: (upper and middle) early and late trophozoites; (lower) meront. The host cells are enlarged and show Schüffner's dots.

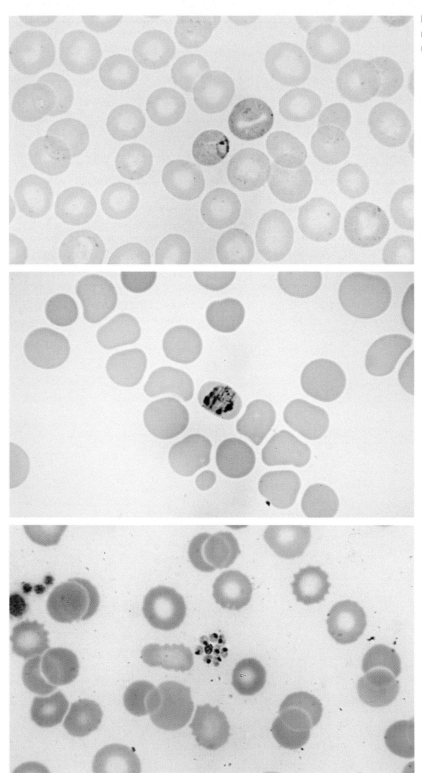

Fig. 1.11 *P. malariae*: (upper and middle) ring and band forms; (lower) meront. Note the malarial pigment.

P. malariae trophozoites are not active and are irregular in shape (Fig. 1.11), often extending across the cell as a band. The infected cell is not enlarged and only rarely shows a few surface dots: Ziemann's dots. The meronts are smaller than those of *P. vivax* (7μm in diameter), and produce only about 6–12 merozoites compared with the 12–24 of *P. vivax* (and 8–24 of *P. falciparum*).

P. ovale resembles *P. malariae* in size and number of merozoites, but the infected cells become enlarged and stippled with Schüffner's dots, like those of *P. vivax*. The cells also seem to lose their rigidity so that they may become distorted and elongated in the preparation of blood films (Fig. 1.12), the feature responsible for the parasite's specific name.

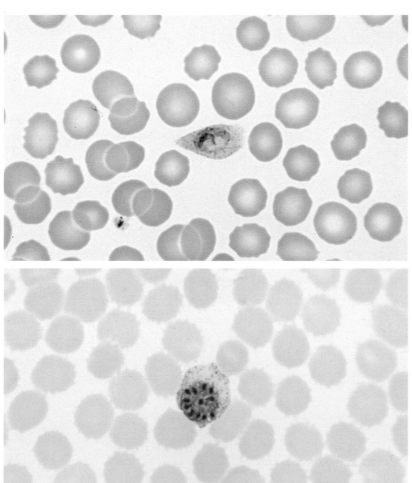

Fig. 1.12 *P. ovale*: (upper) trophozoite; (lower) meront. The host cells may be elongated and show Schüffner's dots.

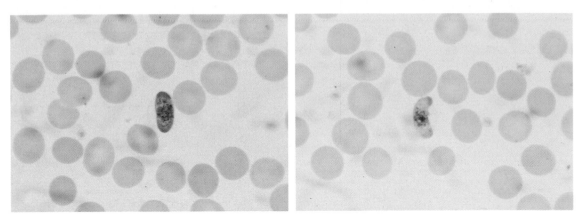

Fig. 1.13   *P. falciparum*: (left) male gametocyte; (right) female gametocyte.

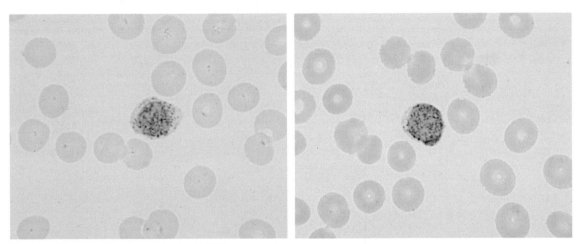

Fig. 1.14   *P. vivax*: (left) male gametocyte; (right) female gametocyte.

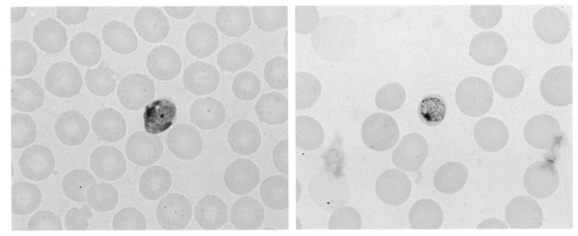

Fig. 1.15   *P. malariae*: (left) male gametocyte; (right) female gametocyte.

This erythrocytic cycle may be repeated or, in response to unknown stimuli, maturation into gametocytes may occur. The male (micro-) and female (macro-) gametocytes of all species can be differentiated as the male has a larger, more diffuse nucleus, in readiness for gamete production after its ingestion by the mosquito; the female has darker staining cytoplasm because it contains numerous ribosomes for protein biosynthesis following fertilization.

P. falciparum gametocytes are crescent-shaped (Fig. 1.13) but those of the other species are spherical (Figs 1.14–1.16).

Cycles of intraerythrocytic merogony continue indefinitely unless terminated by the host's immune response or its death. Merogony in liver cells takes 5.5–15 days, and that in the red blood cells either 48 or 72 hours, depending on the species of *Plasmodium* involved (see below). The developmental cycle in the mosquito vector takes from a week to a month, depending on the ambient temperature: the warmer it is, the quicker the development.

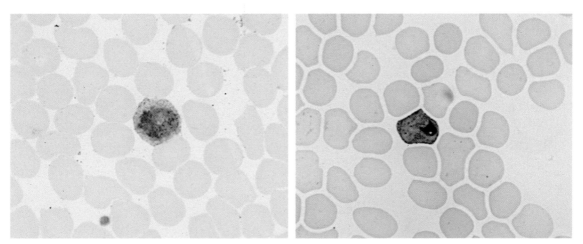

Fig. 1.16 *P. ovale*: (left) male gametocyte; (right) female gametocyte.

Fig. 1.17 Relative sizes of *Plasmodium* gametocytes.

	size of gametocyte	
species	**male**	**female**
P. falciparum	9–11μm	12–14μm
P. vivax	9μm	10–11μm
P. malariae	7μm	7μm
P. ovale	9μm	9μm

One of the characteristics of malaria is the disease's potential for long persistence in infected persons, with characteristic recrudescences or relapses, sometimes after years of subclinical infection.

With *P. vivax* infection, these long term recrudescences may be true relapses, that is, episodes of reinvasion of the blood cells after periods when parasites have been totally absent from the blood, persisting only within liver cells as specialized sporozoites called hypnozoites. The hypnozoites remain dormant within liver cells for varying periods of time until, in response to unknown endogenous or exogenous stimuli, they commence merogony resulting in reinvasion of the erythrocytes by the ensuing merozoites. True relapses of *P. vivax* may occur even after chemotherapy has completely cleared parasites from the peripheral blood, if the drug used is one to which hypnozoites are not sensitive. One subspecies, *P. vivax hibernans*, developed a refinement of this mechanism in which all sporozoites became dormant hypnozoites; consequently, the first clinical attack of malaria was postponed for several months after the infective mosquito bite. This enabled the parasite to overwinter in the cooler, northern regions of its range, where there were no adult mosquitoes available during the winter to ensure transmission before the host's immunity had damped down the parasite population to a level at which its chances of infecting a feeding mosquito were unacceptably reduced. *P. vivax hibernans* persisted in The Netherlands until only a few decades ago, and it was probably this subspecies which occurred in England. Although its range is now more restricted, *P. vivax* still occurs in some temperate regions, notably around the Mediterranean, in the Middle East and in parts of China.

The periodic recrudescences of the other species of *Plasmodium* which infect man result from a small number of erythrocytic parasites which have survived the development of antibodies in the host's plasma, perhaps by being sequestered in circulatory 'backwaters' where antibody concentration remains low, until, after a little-understood process of changing their surface antigens, they are enabled to

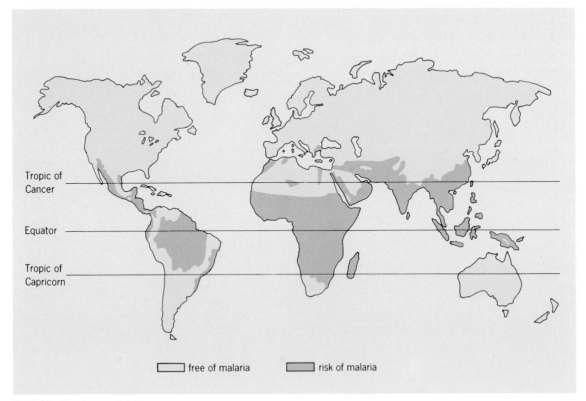

Fig. 1.18 Distribution of malaria.

multiply explosively once again and induce a clinical attack of malaria (compare *Trypanosoma brucei*, p.28).

Malaria in man can occur only where there are susceptible species of mosquito, and where the weather is regularly warm enough for sporogony to be completed within the lifespan of an adult mosquito. In practice, this limits the disease to warmer temperate areas and the subtropics and tropics (Fig. 1.18). *P. vivax* is geographically the most widespread species and in earlier times was common in eastern England. The disappearance of malaria from England was probably the result of increasing living standards, which reduced the close contact between people and *Anopheles* that had existed when country-folk shared accommodation with their domestic animals, on which the mosquitoes also fed, and when farmyards and villages abounded with stagnant water breeding sites for the mosquitoes.

P. falciparum is the commonest species in tropical and subtropical areas, and may sometimes occur in warmer temperate zones. *P. malariae* has a similar range to *P. falciparum* within the tropics and subtropics, but is less common and tends to occur in patches. *P. ovale* is the least common form of human malaria, being almost if not entirely restricted to tropical Africa; there are a few records of its occur-rence in the western Pacific region but some authorities doubt that these infections were actually acquired there or believe that, if they were, they represented merely a chance transmission from another infected person who had brought the parasite from Africa.

Shortly after the end of World War I, there were a few 'casual' transmissions of this kind in England, the organism in these cases being *P. vivax* brought into the country by soldiers returning from endemic areas and transmitted by local mosquitoes, but the parasite did not become re-established in England.

P. malariae is the only malaria parasite of man which can naturally infect another primate, the chimpanzee; it is doubtful, however, if any human infections are derived from mosquitoes infected by feeding on chimpanzees, as contact between man and chimpanzees is not close. Splenectomy renders several types of monkey (including *Macaca* and *Aotus*) susceptible to the other human malarias, which is convenient for research workers. Splenectomized chimpanzees are also susceptible to the other species which infect man.

Clinical effects

The common names for the different forms of malaria are derived from the periodicity of their fevers (Fig. 1.19). Synchronization of the merogony

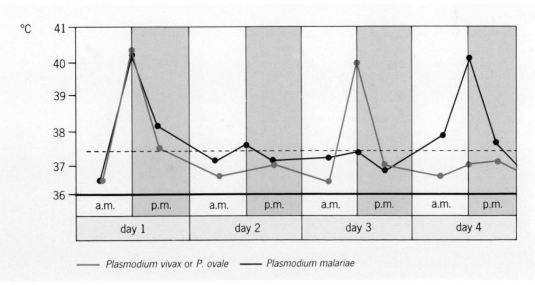

Fig. 1.19 Temperature fluctuations in malaria patients: peaks of fever are related to the intraerythrocytic merogony cycle, occurring every 48 or 72 hours if the cycle is synchronized, as it often is.

cycle leads to rupture of many red cells at once, and the release of proteinaceous debris and malarial pigment causes a peak in fever. If the first day of fever is regarded as day 1, the 72 hour merogony cycle of *P. malariae* leads to another fever peak on day 4 (quartan); the other species peak again on day 3 (tertian).

Because of the destruction of red blood cells caused when meronts rupture, all species of *Plasmodium* cause anaemia. The hepatic meronts do no clinically detectable damage.

Only *P. falciparum* produces disease severe enough to be fatal. This is partly because parasitaemias (numbers of parasites in the blood) tend to be higher and hence the anaemia is more severe, but principally because parasitized erythrocytes adhere to capillary walls and to each other, with the result that small blood vessels become blocked. Their 'stickiness' may be due to the development on their surface of knobs, visible by electron microscopy. Blood vessel blockage leads to anoxia of the vessel endothelium and its rupture. The resulting haemorrhage destroys some of the surrounding tissue; if this occurs in the brain (cerebral malaria) the damage may be severe, even lethal (Figs 1.20–1.22).

Another serious complication of *P. falciparum* infection is blackwater fever: massive intravascular haemolysis results in the excretion of altered haemo-

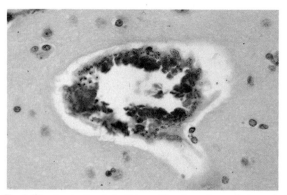
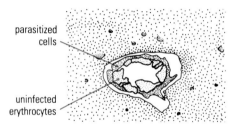

parasitized cells

uninfected erythrocytes

Fig. 1.20 Cerebral malaria. This capillary has a layer of pigmented parasitized cells adhering to its endothelium; the centre contains uninfected (unpigmented) erythrocytes. Adhesion damages the endothelium and uninfected blood cells leak out into the surrounding tissue. H & E stain.

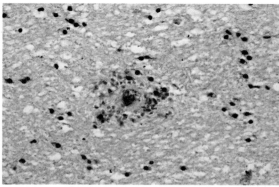
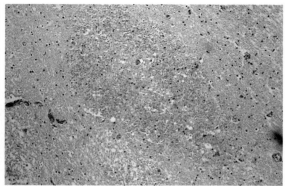

Fig. 1.21 Cerebral malaria. Haemorrhage is at first small (left) but rapidly increases in size (right). H & E stain.

globin in the urine, which is consequently very dark. Blackwater fever is associated with quinine treatment and is therefore now rare; increasing development of drug resistance by *P. falciparum* (see below) is, however, leading to the reuse of quinine, and it is thus possible that this complication may reappear. The haemolysis is thought by some to result from the presence in plasma of free fatty acids which are normally rendered harmless by being bound to plasma proteins; it appears that quinine may interfere with this binding process, leaving the acids free to lyse erythrocytes.

Infection with *P. falciparum* can also lead to abortion if blood sinuses of the placenta become blocked by parasitized cells (Fig. 1.23), depriving the fetus of oxygen and nutrients.

Although the other species of *Plasmodium* which infect man are not considered highly pathogenic, prolonged infection may be very debilitating. There is also evidence that it may cause immunosuppression. It seems that patients with malaria may be predisposed to develop latent viral infections, such as the Epstein–Barr virus associated with infectious mononucleosis, and also to develop Burkitt's lymphoma.

In addition, prolonged infection with *P. malariae* sometimes leads to deposition of antigen–antibody complexes on the glomerular basement membrane in

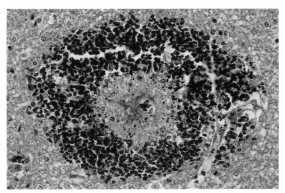
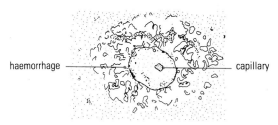

Fig. 1.22 Cerebral malaria. If the patient does not die, phagocytic cells move into the haemorrhage in an attempt to repair the damage. The capillary can still be seen. H & E stain.

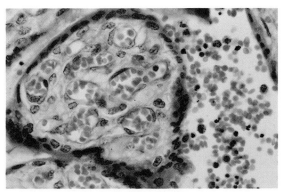
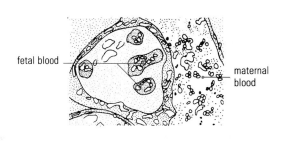

Fig. 1.23 Placenta in *P. falciparum* infection. The maternal blood contains many infected (pigmented) red blood cells, but the blood on the fetal side of the barrier consists of normal, uninfected cells, since the parasites cannot penetrate an undamaged placenta.

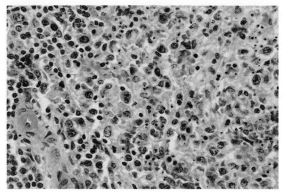

Fig. 1.24 Spleen from a malaria patient. The white pulp (left, stained predominantly blue) contains mainly lymphocytes, and is not obviously affected. The red pulp contains increased numbers of phagocytes and is hyperplastic and engorged with blood. Cells containing parasites are recognizable by dark brown pigment. H & E stain.

the kidney, resulting in serious nephrosis; the full pathogenesis of this is not understood.

The body's mononuclear phagocytic cell system (MPS), of which the spleen is the major aggregation, is very important in the defence against malaria. In persons with malaria the MPS proliferates enormously, and this, in turn, results in gross enlargement of the spleen. Microscopical sections of spleen from malaria patients show that the red pulp, which contains the phagocytic cells, is engorged with blood and with phagocytes (macrophages) containing ingested parasites, recognizable by their contained pigment (Fig. 1.24).

Fig. 1.25 The life cycle of *Toxoplasma gondii.*

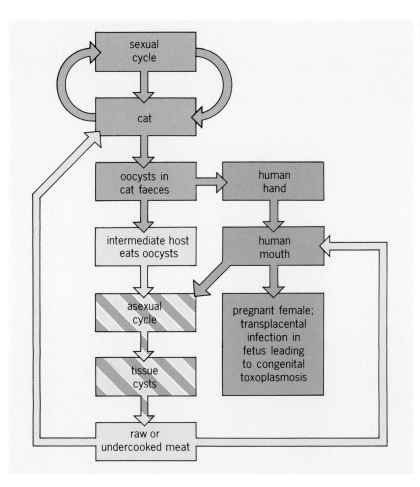

Diagnosis

Although the clinical picture of regularly recurrent fever and splenomegaly suggests malaria, the only sure confirmation is by finding parasites on thick or thin blood films stained with one of the Romanowsky stains, usually Giemsa's, Leishman's or Field's. Serodiagnostic methods are now being used increasingly, particularly for malaria surveys, but are not necessarily indicative of active infection. Suitable tests are indirect immunofluorescence (IFAT), enzyme-linked immunosorbent assay (ELISA) and indirect haemagglutination. IFAT is probably the most sensitive and is best for specific identification, but it has the disadvantage of requiring equipment for fluorescence microscopy.

Treatment

The drugs most commonly used to treat acute malaria are the 4-aminoquinolines, chloroquine and amodiaquine, or quinine. The use of quinine was virtually discontinued because of its association with blackwater fever (see above), but the increasing development of resistance to 4-aminoquinolines by the parasites, especially *P. falciparum*, has led to its reintroduction. In places where resistance is a problem, newer drugs such as mefloquine and/or mixtures of drugs, for example sulfadoxine plus pyrimethamine, are being used. Another new development is the use of *quinghaosu*, also known as artemisin, which is an extract from the plant *Artemisia annua* that has been used as a herbal treatment in China for 2000 years. None of these newer compounds destroys hypnozoites of *P. vivax*; only the intraerythrocytic meronts are affected. Although other drugs relieve a clinical attack of benign tertian malaria, radical cure (prevention of relapses) can be achieved only by the use of primaquine, an 8-aminoquinoline.

Prevention and control

Infection with malaria can be prevented in two ways: either by avoidance of infected mosquito bites, such as by screening windows, spraying inside houses with insecticides and the use of mosquito nets at night; or by the use of prophylactic drugs. A few decades ago suitable prophylactics (for example, proguanil hydrochloride or chloroquine) were almost entirely reliable, but their widespread use (and misuse) has led to the development of resistance by *P. falciparum* on an alarmingly wide scale. It is now very difficult to find entirely reliable, yet non-toxic, prophylactics for use against malaria. Proguanil hydrochloride, taken daily, is very effective but only if parasites in the area concerned are not resistant to it. The same is true of chloroquine, taken weekly, but resistance to chloroquine is the commonest form of resistance, and so it is no longer recommended. Combinations of drugs are being increasingly used, for example pyrimethamine plus sulfadoxine or pyrimethamine plus dapsone. The situation changes almost daily; anyone contemplating travel to a malarious area should seek the latest information from authoritative sources. In the United Kingdom these are the Hospital for Tropical Diseases in London, the Ross Institute (in the London School of Hygiene and Tropical Medicine) and the Liverpool School of Tropical Medicine; in the USA advice can be obtained from the Communicable Diseases Center in Atlanta, Georgia.

Control of malaria is best attempted by anti-mosquito measures (see Chapter 4).

TOXOPLASMA

Causative organism	Disease
Toxoplasma gondii	Toxoplasmosis

Toxoplasma gondii, first described in 1908, was for many years a parasitological enigma which did not seem to fit into any of the available taxonomic groups. In 1971, however, work by Hutchison (in Scotland) and Frenkel (in the USA) showed that it was an apicomplexan, belonging to a group loosely referred to as 'coccidia', many species of which cause economically important disease in chickens. *T. gondii* is dixenous: the definitive host is the domestic cat and a few of its wild relatives; the intermediate host can be any species of mammal or bird (as far as is known). The fact that man may be infected as an intermediate host makes *T. gondii* important in medical parasitology.

Transmission and epidemiology

The life cycle of *T. gondii* is illustrated in Fig. 1.25. Man can become infected with *T. gondii* in several ways: the most important is probably by swallowing oocysts (c.11 × 13μm) passed in the faeces of infected cats (Fig. 1.26). This may occur as a result of children playing in areas which are also used by cats as defaecation sites, or as a result of handling domestic pets and not being scrupulously careful about hand-washing afterwards. Other routes of infection are by eating raw or undercooked meat of an animal which has been an intermediate host and which contains viable parasites. Of great clinical importance is transplacental infection of the fetus from a mother with an acute infection of toxoplasmosis.

T. gondii is a very successful parasite; it has a wide geographical distribution and serological evidence shows that about one quarter of the adult population of the UK, USA and many other countries are or have been infected.

In some areas, much higher rates have been recorded, for example 94 per cent in Guatemala. Fortunately, infection with *Toxoplasma* is usually asymptomatic or causes only mild illness (except in the infected fetus). In spite of its prevalence in the UK, fewer than 200 cases of recognizable disease result annually, and naturally infected cats are rarely, if ever, ill. This good adaptation of parasite to host is part of the success of *T. gondii*; it seldom kills its hosts. *T. gondii* is equally or more common in its non-human hosts: surveys of cats have indicated a prevalence of around 77 per cent; 32 per cent has been reported for dogs, 21 per cent for cattle, 50 per cent for pigs, and 64 per cent for sheep. The com-

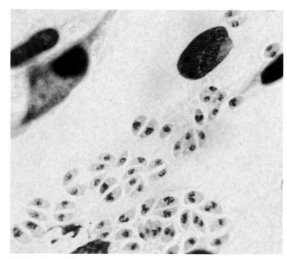

Fig. 1.26 Infective sporulated oocysts of *T. gondii* in cat faeces. Courtesy of Prof. W M Hutchison.

Fig. 1.27 Tachyzoites of *T. gondii* liberated from ruptured pseudocysts. Giemsa's stain.

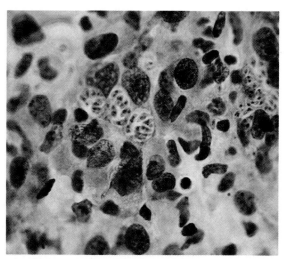

Fig. 1.28 Intracellular groups (pseudocysts) of *T. gondii* tachyzoites in smear of mouse peritoneal fluid. Giemsa's stain.

mon presence of farm cats in barns, byres and feedstores presumably accounts for the high infection rates in domestic herbivores.

Swallowing the oocyst initiates the extraintestinal asexual cycle of development, which occurs mainly in macrophages. This is the only part of the cycle which occurs in intermediate hosts. The sporozoites, emerging from the ingested oocyst in the small intestine, pass through the mucosa and are phagocytosed by, or actively enter, macrophages. In the macrophage the lysosomes are inhibited from fusion with the phagosomes and the parasites contained in them thus are not killed by the lysosomal enzymes. The parasites in this phase of development are called tachyzoites (from the Greek *tachos*, speed, because they divide rapidly) or endozoites and measure c.5 × 1–2μm. They divide until they fill the host cell, which then liberates them (Fig. 1.27), and they reinvade (or are ingested by) other macrophages, repeating the process. The cell which contains them, when it becomes merely a bag full of tachyzoites, is called a pseudocyst (Fig. 1.28). These events constitute the acute phase of infection. If the host lives, and the infection is untreated, the host's immune system becomes effective and tachyzoites are destroyed, presumably at the vulnerable stage of passing from cell to cell. However, the parasite responds to this by entering other cells (muscle cells, neurons, and perhaps others) and secreting a thin but tough cyst wall around itself. Within this cyst, which can measure up to 60μm in diameter, protected from the host's antibodies, the parasites multiply slowly, and hence are now known as bradyzoites (Greek *brady*, slow) or cystozoites (Figs 1.29 & 1.30).

If another intermediate host eats uncooked meat containing these tissue cysts, the bradyzoites emerge in the duodenum and repeat the extraintestinal cycle. However, if a non-immune cat ingests tissue cysts (or tachyzoites) in infected prey (or raw meat and offal fed to it), the emerging bradyzoites (or the tachyzoites) enter cells of the duodenal mucosa and begin the intestinal cycle of development, which occurs only in the definitive host. This cycle consists of a limited number of merogonies, producing merozoites which reinvade other mucosal cells, until the final generation of merozoites enter mucosal cells

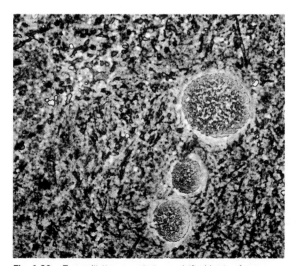

Fig. 1.29 *T. gondii:* tissue cysts in emulsified brain of mouse. Phase contrast illumination. Courtesy of Prof. W M Hutchison.

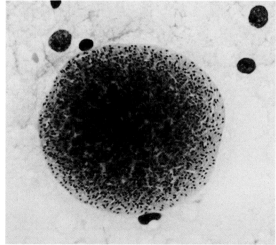

Fig. 1.30 Large tissue cyst of *T. gondii* in emulsified brain. Individual bradyzoites are visible around the periphery. Giemsa's stain.

and commence the sexual cycle of gametogony, fertilization and sporogony within the developing oocyst (Figs 1.31–1.34). The cycle is basically like that of *Plasmodium*, but the host cells differ.

The oocyst, a thick-walled resistant structure (c. 10 × 12μm), is liberated from the intestinal epithelial cell while still immature; it completes its development while passing down the gut and after expulsion in the faeces. Its contents divide first into two cells; these then secrete cyst walls to form two sporocysts. The contents of each sporocyst then divide once more to produce two infective sporozoites. Once mature, the oocyst may infect any warm-blooded animal which swallows it. The sporozoites are liberated, through digestion of the oocyst and sporocyst walls, in the small intestine, penetrate the mucosa and enter macrophages in which they initiate the extraintestinal cycle of asexual development.

In the definitive host, invasion of the intestinal mucosa and subsequent merogony and gametogony apparently does not always occur after ingestion of oocysts or tachyzoites but almost always does so after infection with tissue cysts and bradyzoites, unless the cat is immune. From the point of view of the epidemiology of human infection, the oocyst is the most significant stage, since its thick, resistant wall enables it to survive for a year or more.

Clinical effects

• Postnatal toxoplasmosis

Infection with *T. gondii* usually gives rise to a mild disease, characterized by fever and enlargement of the lymph glands. It may be so mild as to pass unnoticed or may produce a mild fever and be mistaken for 'flu'. Sometimes, for example in immunocompromised persons, intense generalized infection develops, with tachyzoites proliferating throughout brain, lungs, liver and elsewhere; such infections may be fatal. If death does not ensue and if the infection is not adequately treated, the initial acute phase (when tachyzoite multiplication occurs) passes into the chronic phase, characterized by the presence of bradyzoites in tissue cysts only. The chronic phase is symptomless, and may persist for many years — perhaps for the lifetime of the patient.

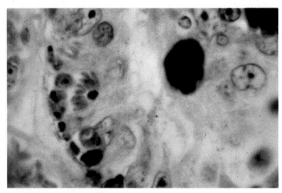

Fig. 1.31 Fan-shaped array of merozoites in meront of *T. gondii*, within epithelial cell of small intestine of cat. Courtesy of Prof. W M Hutchison.

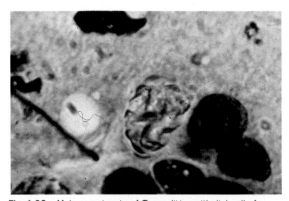

Fig. 1.32 Male gametocyte of *T. gondii* in epithelial cell of small intestine of cat. The developing, curved microgametes (c. 5μm long) can be seen, but their flagella are not obvious. Courtesy of Prof. W M Hutchison.

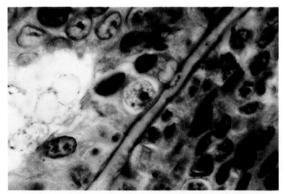

Fig. 1.33 Female gametocyte of *T. gondii* in gut epithelial cell; it measures c. 7–8μm in diameter. Courtesy of Prof. W M Hutchison.

It is presumed that tissue cysts rupture at intervals, some of the bradyzoites evading the host's antibodies by rapidly entering other nearby cells and re-encysting. Tissue cysts commonly occur in the brain (Fig. 1.35), where they do no obvious damage.

• Congenital toxoplasmosis

Infection *in utero* with *T. gondii* is relatively rare, with an incidence probably below one per 1000 live births, but it may cause severe damage to, and even death of, the fetus. Intense proliferation of tachyzoites in the brain damages large areas and may cause death. Infants who survive may be born with hydrocephalus and often die soon after birth. Less severely affected fetuses may be born blind or with less severe retinal damage.

Diagnosis

Suspected toxoplasmosis may be confirmed by isolation of the parasite in tonsil or lymph gland biopsy and inoculation into mice. There are several serological tests, but positivity indicates only that the person has been infected at some time and may now be chronically infected. However, if two tests are done with an interval of a few weeks, and the second gives a significantly higher titre of antibodies than the first, it is likely that the patient is acutely infected. Tests which are used include CF,agglutination, IFAT and the *Toxoplasma* dye test, which depends on the fact that tachyzoites (from experimentally infected mice) mixed with specific antibody and complement do not stain with methylene blue. The dye test is less commonly used now, as its dependence on live tachyzoites makes it hazardous for the technician, and it is being supplanted by the other tests which use dead parasites as antigen.

Treatment

Acute postnatal toxoplasmosis can be treated with a mixture of pyrimethamine and sulphonamides or, if this is contraindicated because the patient is pregnant, with spiramycin. The damage caused by transplacental infection cannot be reversed.

Prevention and control

Prevention is simple in theory but difficult in practice: it consists of avoiding the ingestion of oocysts or tissue cysts. This can be done by never eating raw or undercooked meat, by washing hands and instruments thoroughly after preparing raw meat, and by avoiding cats, especially their handling. The rarity of clinical infection in adults, and its customary mildness, suggest that it may not be worth going to great lengths to avoid infection. It may, however, be worthwhile preventing cats from defaecating in children's play areas, for example, by covering them when not in use.

The severity of congenital infection means that pregnant women should, perhaps, be rather more careful. Infection of the fetus occurs only if the mother has an acute attack while pregnant, not if she is chronically infected, so, ideally, a serological test

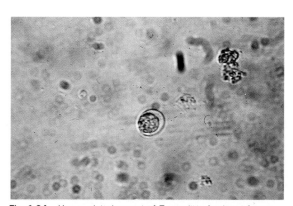

Fig. 1.34 Unsporulated oocyst of *T. gondii* in fresh cat faeces. Courtesy of Prof. W M Hutchison.

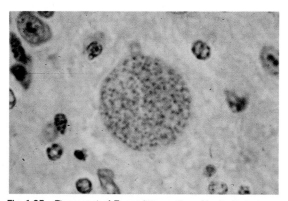

Fig. 1.35 Tissue cyst of *T. gondii* in section of brain; there is no obvious reaction or damage to tissue around the cyst. Courtesy of Prof. W M Hutchison.

should be done in early pregnancy. If negative, the woman should be advised to be particularly careful about handling and eating raw meat, and should perhaps avoid too much contact with the household cat. However, since routine testing for anti-*Toxoplasma* antibodies is not done in the UK, this is really a counsel of perfection. Another possibility would be to examine the cat's faeces for oocysts and treat the animal; but this, too, is rather impractical.

SARCOCYSTIS

Causative organisms	Disease
Sarcocystis bovihominis	Sarcocystosis
S. suihominis, possibly other species	

Sarcocystis is closely related to *Toxoplasma* but differs in not having a wide range of intermediate hosts. The extraintestinal phase, which does not develop in the final, definitive host, occurs in muscle cells. These may be transformed into large cysts (Fig. 1.36), in some species several millimetres in length, containing 'zoites' which, while similar to those of *Toxoplasma*, are bigger (10–15μm long; Fig. 1.37). The extraintestinal phase is usually symptomless, unless infections are abnormally heavy. The intestinal phase, also similar to that of *Toxoplasma*, may be symptomless or may cause fairly severe, though usually self-limiting, diarrhoea; treatment is not usually given.

Man is the definitive host of at least two species, *S. bovihominis* and *S. suihominis*, of which the intermediate hosts are oxen and pigs, respectively. The nomenclature of *Sarcocystis* species is a matter of some controversy at present, as its full life cycle and dependence on two hosts have become known only relatively recently. There are a few older records of human infection with the muscle cysts ('sarcocysts'), indicating that man can, sometimes, act as intermediate host for species with unidentified definitive hosts; such infections are so rare that it is likely that they represent aberrant, accidental infections rather than part of a normal life cycle.

The organism known as *Isospora belli*, which has been rarely reported as causing mild diarrhoea in humans, may turn out to be merely a stage in the life cycle of another species of *Sarcocystis*.

BABESIA

Causative organism	Disease
Babesia divergens	European human babesiosis
Babesia microti	American human babesiosis

Babesia species are apicomplexans, commonly known as 'piroplasms'; they are fairly closely related to *Plasmodium* and do not normally infect man. They, and the closely related genus *Theileria*, are common causes of disease in cattle, sheep and horses in many parts of the world, and also infect a wide range of wild animals.

Babesia (only 1–2μm long) inhabits erythrocytes in its mammalian host (Fig. 1.38), in which it multiplies only by binary fission, causing a disease characterized by fever and anaemia, not unlike malaria. Some species, including *B. microti*, have a single cycle of merogony within lymphocytes before invasion of the red cells occurs. All species are transmitted by invertebrate vector hosts which are always ticks (Arthropoda, Acarina) and almost always members of the family Ixodidae, the 'hard' ticks.

There have been rare reports of human infection with *Babesia* spp.; fewer than fifty cases have been reported though some may have been misdiagnosed as malaria. In North America, these are due to *B. microti*, a species which is normally restricted to voles (*Microtus* spp.), giving rise to relatively benign malaria-like episodes which have resolved spontaneously. In Europe, a few human infections have been recorded in splenectomized persons; almost all have been fatal, and some (probably all) have been caused by *B. divergens*, which normally infects cattle. No successful treatment has been found for human babesiosis.

PNEUMOCYSTIS

Causative organism	Disease
Pneumocystis carinii	Atypical interstitial plasma cell pneumonia

Pneumocystis carinii is an organism of uncertain, and disputed, taxonomic position; it is probably an apicomplexan protozoon, but has been regarded as a fungus or even a modified mitochondrion of the affected person's pneumocytes. It occurs in man, dogs and rodents in the Americas, Europe, Australia, China and possibly elsewhere.

Transmission is presumably by droplet infection; chronically infected adults or, possibly, dogs or rodents may serve as reservoirs of infection.

Although perhaps a fairly common inhabitant of the human lung, *P. carinii* rarely causes disease; it is particularly prone to do this in immunocompromised persons such as weak or premature babies, persons on immunosuppressive therapy, or those afflicted

with the acquired immunodeficiency syndrome (AIDS). The organisms, which are about 5–6μm in diameter, live extracellularly in the lung alveolae. When sufficiently numerous to be pathogenic, they cause the alveolae to become blocked with a mass of parasites and plasma cells, embedded in mucus (Fig. 1.39). The resulting pneumonia is non-febrile and does not respond to conventional antibiotic therapy. Treatment with pentamidine, or sulphonamide-diaminopyrimidine mixtures such as sulphamethoxazole plus trimethoprim (co-trimoxazole), has had some success.

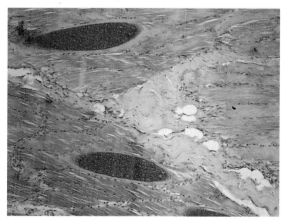

Fig. 1.36 Sarcocysts of *S. 'lindemanni'* in human muscle.

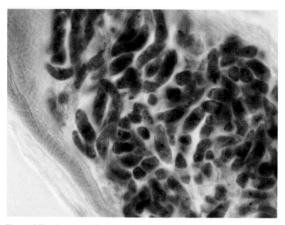

Fig. 1.37 Zoites of *S. muris* within a sarcocyst.

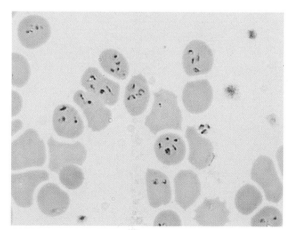

Fig. 1.38 *Babesia divergens* in erythrocytes of an ox; small, pear-shaped organisms (from which the term 'piroplasm' was derived). Courtesy of Dr A D Irvin.

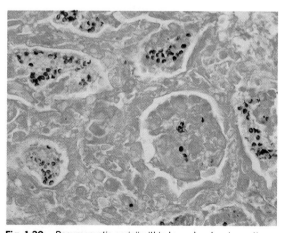

Fig. 1.39 *Pneumocystis carinii* within lung alveolae, in section. Parasites are darkly stained with Grocott's silver stain and contrast well with the background of methyl green-stained lung cells and alveolae filled with plasma cells and mucus.

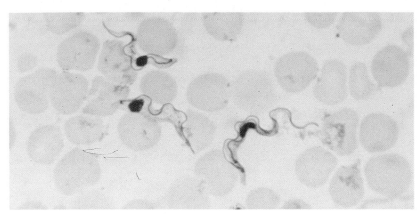

Fig. 1.40 *Trypanosoma brucei*: haematozoic trypomastigotes in mouse blood. Note the anterior flagellum, which runs along the side of the cell forming the undulating membrane; the typical trypomastigote form has the flagellar origin (basal body) at the posterior end of the cell, where the kinetoplast lies. The central nucleus can also be seen. Giemsa's stain.

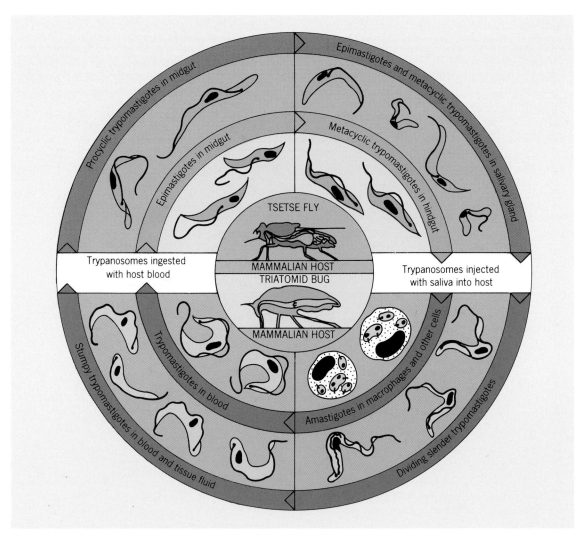

Fig. 1.41 The life cycle of *Trypanosoma brucei* (outer circle) and *T. cruzi* (inner circle).

TRYPANOSOMA

Trypanosomes are elongated organisms with a single flagellum. They have one special feature, an unusually large amount of mitochondrial DNA; this is aggregated into a single mass one to several micrometres in length (the kinetoplast), and is easily visible by light microscopy (Fig. 1.40). The life cycle of *Trypanosoma* is illustrated in Fig. 1.41.

Causative organism	Disease
Trypanosoma brucei	African human
Trypanosoma brucei gambiense	trypanosomiasis or
	sleeping sickness

The nomenclature of *Trypanosoma brucei* is confused. Originally, in the early years of this century, three African species were named: *T. brucei*, which was believed to be unable to infect man; *T. rhodesiense*, which could infect man, in whom it caused an acute disease; and *T. gambiense*, also infective to man but producing a much more chronic disease. It was later realized that the three 'species' were closely related, and they were reduced to subspecies of *T. brucei*; *T. b. brucei*, *T. b. gambiense* and *T. b. rhodesiense*.

The most popular view at present is that the erstwhile *T. gambiense* is a subspecies of *T. brucei*, while *T. rhodesiense* is nothing more than a collection of strains of *T. brucei* that have the property of acquiring, and perhaps losing, the ability to resist the potentially trypanosomicidal effect of human plasma.

Transmission and epidemiology

T. brucei is transmitted by tsetse flies, large blood-sucking Diptera of the genus *Glossina*. Unlike mosquitoes, both sexes of *Glossina* feed exclusively on blood, so that both can transmit trypanosomes. *Glossina* is restricted to tropical Africa, which is the reason for the similar restriction of *T. brucei* (Fig. 1.42). Curiously, most tsetse flies seem to be resistant to infection with the trypanosomes, and under natural conditions usually fewer than 1 per cent are infected. Once infected, however, a fly remains infective for life.

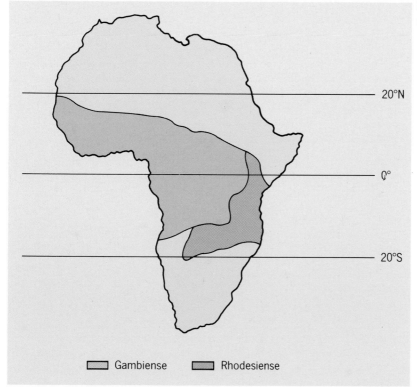

Fig. 1.42 The distribution of African human trypanosomiasis.

20°N

0°

20°S

☐ Gambiense   ☐ Rhodesiense

In the insect, the trypanosomes undergo a complicated developmental cycle, some details of which are still obscure. Parasites ingested in blood from an infected mammal develop first in the insect's midgut. They elongate into procyclic forms (Fig. 1.43) and multiply by binary fission; at this stage they are contained within the peritrophic membrane, a chitinous inner tube which lines the fly's midgut. They then migrate into the space between the membrane and the gut wall, where they are safe from expulsion with the digested blood as it is passed back into the hindgut and eventually voided as faeces.

In those flies which are destined to become infective, parasites invade the salivary glands. There is still some doubt about the route by which they do this. Once in the salivary glands, they transform into epimastigotes (Fig. 1.44). These become attached to the lining of the glands, by means of balloon-like expansions of the tips of their flagella, and continue to divide by binary fission.

Two to three weeks after the infective feed, the epimastigotes become free in the lumen of the salivary gland and undergo transformation into metacyclic trypomastigotes (Fig. 1.45). These infective forms are injected with the fly's saliva into the next mammal on which it feeds.

The metacyclic forms within the fly acquire a glycoprotein coat on the outer surface of the cell membrane. This coat is also present on the trypomastigotes developing in the mammalian host and host lymphocytes produce antibodies to the coat protein. With the aid of complement, the parasites are lysed. The trypanosomes change the molecular arrangement of the coat repeatedly, at fairly regular intervals, however, and thus avoid destruction of the whole population. The host's immune system fails to recognize individuals with the altered surface; these survive and continue multiplication. Parasitaemia thus proceeds in a series of waves, each successive variant antigenic type increasing in number until the host has synthesized the appropriate antibody. The process is repeated many times, until the host is either successfully treated or dies; perhaps, rarely, the infection may be eliminated. The synthesis of the successive variant surface glycoproteins is under genetic control; although it does not occur in a fixed sequence, it is not entirely random. Details of the control of the process of antigenic variation are not yet fully known. The subject is very complex, and more information can be obtained from some of the suggested further reading.

After injection into a susceptible mammalian host, the metacyclic trypomastigotes change into the more elongated bloodstream, or haematozoic, forms and divide by binary fission. The parasites do not enter any cells but are at first restricted to the subcutaneous tissue fluid around the site of the fly bite. The host's inflammatory response to the parasites usually results in a localized, tender reddish swelling, the chancre.

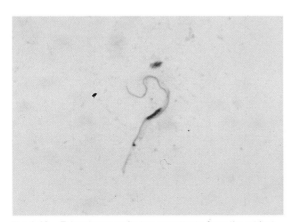

Fig. 1.43 *T. brucei*: procyclic trypomastigote from the midgut of a tsetse fly. Note the posterior extension of the cell, behind the kinetoplast. Giemsa's stain.

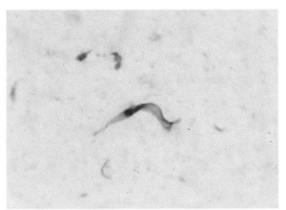

Fig. 1.44 *T. brucei*: epimastigote from tsetse salivary gland. Epimastigotes are characterized by having the flagellar basal body and kinetoplast close to the nucleus in the centre of the cell. Giemsa's stain.

During the next few days the parasites spread throughout the host's lymphatic and blood systems. *T. b. gambiense*, in particular, may be more plentiful in lymphatics and lymph glands than it is in circulating blood. After a variable time (weeks or months with the acute 'rhodesiense'-type infection and months or even years with the chronic *T. b. gambiense* disease), the trypanosomes penetrate into the central nervous system (CNS). Here, too, they remain extracellular.

The trypanosomes which divide in the mammalian host are long slender individuals, about 30 × 1.5μm, with a long flagellum that extends beyond the anterior end of the cell. After a few days, shorter, more stumpy forms develop (Fig. 1.46), about 18μm long and 3–4μm wide, with the flagellum extending only very little, if at all, beyond the anterior end of the cell. These stumpy forms, which do not divide in the mammalian host, are those destined to continue the life cycle after being ingested by a tsetse fly, in which they elongate into the procyclic forms described above. The slender trypomastigotes cannot survive in the vector's gut.

Until recently it was accepted that there was no sexual phase in the life cycle of *T. brucei*. There is now indirect evidence that genetic exchange can occur during development in the vector; such exchange has not been visualized, however. It seems likely that this occurs only rarely and that it depends on the coming together of partners of appropriate 'mating type', strain or population. Chromosomal analysis has shown that the haematozoic stages are diploid.

T. brucei can infect a wide range of mammals and it can produce a very low-grade infection in chickens. In practice, ungulates are the most important hosts from the point of view of human infection, as they may form significant reservoirs of potentially infective strains. In East Africa, domestic cattle and wild antelope are the more important reservoir hosts; transmission to man is usually via *Glossina morsitans* or *G. pallidipes*, species which can survive under relatively dry conditions and inhabit vast areas of East African savanna plains. Consequently human trypanosomiasis in East Africa is often acquired by hunters and travellers in areas infested with these species of tsetse fly, rather than being a predominantly peridomestic infection.

In West and Central Africa, however, where *T. b. gambiense* predominates, it appears that domestic pigs are the most important animal reservoir, although the parasite has also been isolated from wild antelope. Transmission is mainly via *G. palpalis* and closely related species, which need a more humid environment and so are usually restricted to the shores of rivers and lakes. Infections of *T. b. gambiense* in West and Central Africa are therefore characteristically acquired at river crossings, or at watering and washing places in or near villages. Women and children are therefore more likely to be infected with this subspecies than they are with the rhodesiense form.

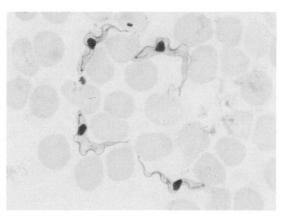

Fig. 1.45 *T. brucei*: metacyclic trypomastigotes from tsetse salivary gland. Giemsa's stain.

Fig. 1.46 *T. brucei*: stumpy haematozoic trypomastigotes in blood of a mouse; some stumpy forms have a posteriorly placed nucleus. Giemsa's stain.

Clinical effects

T. b. gambiense and 'rhodesiense' can be discussed together here, since the type of disease they produce differs quantitatively but not qualitatively. In the early stage of the disease, after development of the chancre, infection of the blood and lymph system results in a more or less acute febrile illness. Infected lymph glands, especially those at the back of the neck, may become very enlarged; the swollen cervical glands constitute 'Winterbottom's sign', a classical diagnostic indication of infection with *T. b. gambiense*. This stage of the illness is rarely, if ever, fatal. More serious effects result from the penetration of the parasites into the CNS, which may occur at any time from weeks ('rhodesiense') to years (*T. b. gambiense*) after initial infection. Here the parasites multiply in the blood vessels, tissue fluids, and cerebrospinal fluid (CSF).

The infected host responds by mounting a cellular and humoral immune reaction. Immunoglobulin (IgM) is secreted into the CSF (as it is in the blood during the early stage), and there is massive infiltration of lymphocytes into the membrane covering the brain, especially the arachnoid membrane and the pia mater. Since the pia mater surrounds all the blood vessels in the brain, its thickening and the lymphocytic infiltrate appear as characteristic 'perivascular cuffing' within the brain substance (Fig. 1.47).

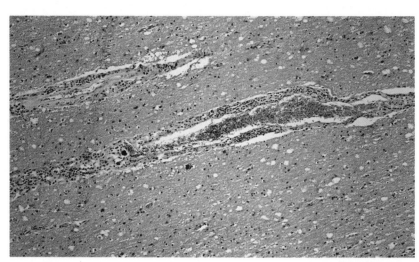

Fig. 1.47 Lymphocytic cell infiltration ('perivascular cuffing') around a small blood vessel in a section of the brain of a patient who died from *T. brucei* infection. H & E stain.

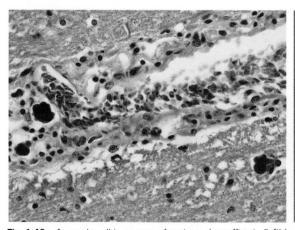
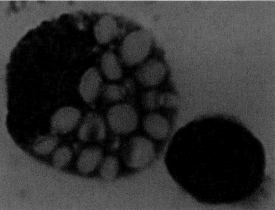

Fig. 1.48 A morula cell in an area of perivascular cuffing in (left) brain section (H & E stain) and (right) in a Giemsa-stained smear of cerebrospinal fluid.

Among the infiltrating cells are 'mulberry-like' bodies, the morula (or Mott) cells (Fig. 1.48); these are plasma cells in the final stage of immunoglobulin secretion.

The outcome of the inflammatory process (meningoencephalitis) is brain damage leading to somnolence, coma and, unless treated, death in almost all cases. A few records exist of healthy carriers who, although infected and with trypanosomes in their blood, appear to remain well and do not develop the late stage of the disease.

Diagnosis

A preliminary diagnosis may be based on clinical signs and symptoms, including the chancre if the patient is seen early enough, and a history of exposure to tsetse bites in an area where the disease is endemic.

A variety of immunological tests may also be used, including IFAT, CF, agglutination and ELISA. A card agglutination test (CAT) is commercially available: plastic-coated cards contain particles of antigen (either killed parasites, or red blood cells or other particles coated with antigen) in wells to which serum is added; if antibody is present, the particles clump together visibly. African trypanosomiasis characteristically results in a marked increase in the amount of IgM in the plasma, and detection of this by immunodiffusion tests can suggest, but not confirm, infection.

Confirmatory diagnosis can be made only by demonstrating the parasites. This can be attempted either microscopically or by inoculation to laboratory rats or mice; cultivation *in vitro* is difficult and rarely tried. In the early stage of infection, blood or lymph gland exudate is examined; in the late stage, CSF is obtained by lumbar puncture. *T. b. gambiense* is more difficult to isolate than 'rhodesiense', as parasites are more scanty in the blood and do not so readily infect laboratory rodents. Therefore, puncture of an enlarged lymph gland may be more fruitful than taking blood, and, if animal inoculation is to be used, it is better to use very young (unweaned) rats if possible. If the CNS has been invaded, CSF will contain (in addition to trypanosomes, which may be very scanty) many more lymphocytes than normal (more than 5 cells/mm^3), morula cells and IgM.

Treatment

In the early stage of infection, before CNS involvement has occurred, African human trypanosomiasis is usually treated with suramin; the drug is fairly effective but is toxic to some patients. Pentamidine is sometimes used for *T. b. gambiense* infection, and occasionally for prophylactic use against this subspecies, but this usage carries a risk of suppressing the clinical disease until the CNS has been invaded, when treatment is more difficult. Prophylaxis against 'rhodesiense' infection is not recommended.

After parasites have entered the CNS, the only effective treatment (and it is not always effective) is the arsenical drug melarsen oxide/BAL or Mel B. Melarsen oxide is a very toxic compound and must be given under strict medical supervision. BAL, or B, stands for British anti-lewisite, an antidote for the chemical warfare gas lewisite, which is given in the hope of reducing the toxicity of melarsen oxide. Patients who do not respond to treatment with Mel B are sometimes given nitrofurazone.

Prevention and control

Prevention involves avoiding being bitten by flies in endemic areas; this may be difficult as tsetse flies are daytime feeders and very persistent, may be very numerous and can bite through thin clothing such as a cotton shirt. As so few flies are infective (fewer than 1 per cent, see above), the chance of being infected is low unless one is exposed repeatedly to bites. As mentioned above, drug prophylaxis is of doubtful value and is never used against 'rhodesiense' infection.

Control of the disease is almost always attempted by controlling, or exterminating, the vectors. Since, especially in East Africa, the tsetse flies inhabit very large areas, their control is difficult. Insecticidal spraying is most cost-effective against the vectors of *T. b. gambiense*, which have more restricted habitats. Aerial spraying is sometimes used but is expensive.

Another approach, also expensive and ecologically destructive, is to remove the tsetse flies' habitat by vegetational clearing (bush clearing); to some extent this can be done selectively.

A third line of attack is by trapping flies, often using traps impregnated with insecticide so that insects merely alighting on the trap are killed. Trapping has become more predominant since it was

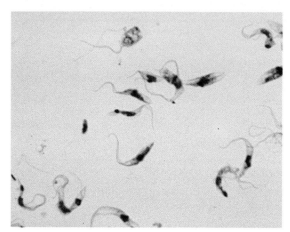

Fig. 1.49 Epimastigotes and metacyclic trypomastigotes of *T. cruzi* from the gut of an infected kissing bug. Giemsa's stain.

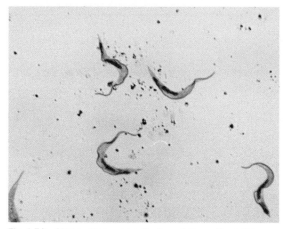

Fig. 1.50 Metacyclic trypomastigotes of *T. cruzi* from the faeces of a kissing bug. Giemsa's stain.

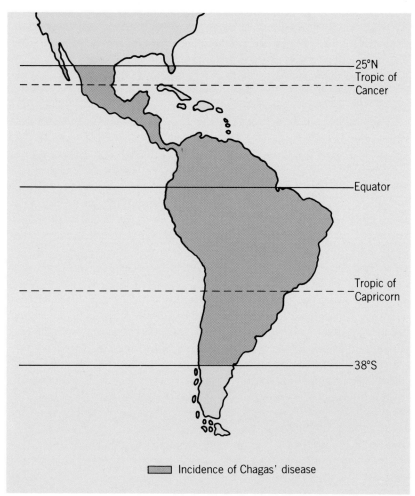

Fig. 1.51 Map of Central and South America, showing distribution of Chagas' disease.

discovered that baiting traps with certain chemicals, which occur naturally in breath and secretions of oxen, greatly increases the number of flies caught.

Causative organism	Disease
Trypanosoma cruzi	South American human trypanosomiasis; Chagas' disease

Transmission and epidemiology

Trypanosoma cruzi is transmitted by 'kissing bugs' (so named because they often feed around the lips of sleeping people), large insects of the family Reduviidae (Hemiptera), subfamily Triatominae. Both sexes feed exclusively on blood.

The development of *T. cruzi* in the bugs is restricted to the gut. The haematozoic trypomastigotes ingested with the blood meal change into epimastigotes (Fig. 1.49) in the insect's midgut and undergo binary fission. They are passed back down the gut with the blood meal which is being digested, and when they reach the hindgut they transform into small metacyclic trypomastigotes which, like those of *T. brucei*, do not divide (Fig. 1.50). These metacyclic trypomastigotes are voided when the bug defaecates, which it does immediately after, or while, feeding. The trypanosomes penetrate the host's skin through the puncture made by the bug's proboscis and initiate infection if the host is susceptible. The bugs usually feed indoors at night; a half-awakened person, especially a child, may scratch the site of the bite and then rub their eyes, transferring parasites to the conjunctiva which they can penetrate.

T. cruzi can infect many, perhaps all, species of mammal but not other animals. Consequently domestic dogs or cats may act as reservoir hosts, as may rodents and other wild animals that live near human habitation and on which bugs feed, such as armadilloes, opossums, racoons and vampire bats. The disease, which affects millions of people throughout South and Central America (Fig. 1.51), is essentially one of poverty. The vector bugs live in cracks in mud-walled houses and similar places, so that persons wealthy enough to have well maintained, high-standard housing are at very little risk of infection.

Once in a susceptible mammal, the metacyclic trypomastigotes, actively or by phagocytosis, enter cells, including macrophages and muscle cells. Within the cells, they transform into small, rounded organisms c. 4μm in diameter, with, at best, a very short flagellum (Fig. 1.52). These forms multiply by binary fission until they fill the host cell, which is then ruptured to release trypomastigotes into the bloodstream and disseminate the infection to other

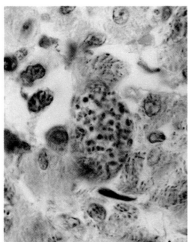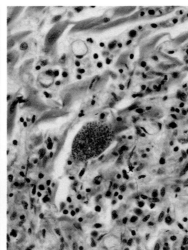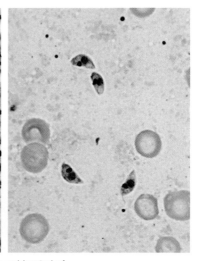

Fig. 1.52 Amastigotes of *T. cruzi* within sections of cardiac muscle cell of (left) a mouse and (centre) of a human patient, H & E stain; (right) amastigotes in a smear from an experimentally infected mouse. Giemsa's stain.

parts of the body. The haematozoic trypomastigotes are smaller than those of *T. brucei*, being about 20μm long; they have a pointed posterior end and are often curved into a C-shape (Fig. 1.53). They do not divide, but enter other host cells to restart the cycle of intracellular multiplication after transforming into amastigotes.

Unlike *T. brucei*, *T. cruzi* does not have a dense surface coat, nor does it undergo antigenic variation; the parasites presumably survive the host's antigenic attack by rapidly escaping from the blood to an intracellular sanctuary. Once inside cells, they are protected from antibody. They survive even in macrophages, cells which digest phagocytosed microorganisms; by escaping from the phagosome into the cytoplasm, before the phagosome fuses with lysosomes and thus avoiding exposure to digestive enzymes.

The haematozoic trypanosomes of *T. cruzi* are not sharply divided into two morphological forms, though some workers believe that slender trypomastigotes which are destined to re-enter cells can be distinguished from broader forms which serve to infect the next hungry kissing bug. There is no evidence of genetic exchange in this species.

T. cruzi, in contrast to *T. brucei*, infects a very high proportion of the bug population, usually more than 50 per cent and sometimes up to 100 per cent.

Clinical effects

Chagas' disease is a chronic condition. Infected persons may show few, if any, signs of disease and may survive for decades, even though still infected.

The first sign of infection may be a swelling at the site of the bite, analogous to a chancre, called a chagoma. If infection occurs via the conjunctiva, a unilateral chagoma involving the eye, and called Romaña's sign, may develop. A more or less acute, febrile illness which is rarely fatal may follow. The disease then settles down into its chronic phase.

During the chronic phase, although signs may not be apparent, the repeated cycles of intracellular multiplication are continually destroying cells, not only those in which the amastigotes multiply, but also neighbouring cells. An autoimmune mechanism is probably involved. Neurons are particularly vulnerable to destruction. If the intracellular groups of parasites (pseudocysts) are concentrated in parts of the gastrointestinal tract, especially the oesophagus or colon, peristalsis may be interfered with and the organ may become hugely distended. This condition is indicated by the prefix mega; for example mega-oesophagus or megacolon. The unfortunate patient may be unable to swallow and so may die of starvation. Megacolon may become so gross as to lead to rupture of the colon and death.

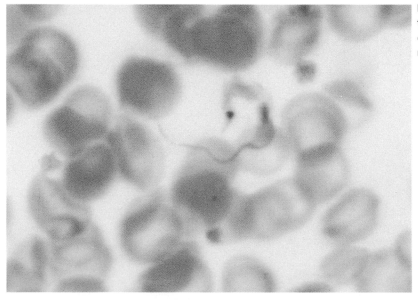

Fig. 1.53 Haematozoic trypomastigote of *T. cruzi* in blood of an experimentally infected mouse. Giemsa's stain.

If the pseudocysts congregate in the heart muscle, and some strains are more prone to do this than others, the ensuing neuronal and muscle cell destruction may gravely weaken the heart wall, causing irreversible damage and leading to an early death from heart attack (Fig. 1.54).

Diagnosis

Clinical signs can only be suggestive, as can immunological tests; IFAT, ELISA and CF are all used. Confirmatory diagnosis by parasite demonstration is easier than for *T. brucei*. Although *T. cruzi* parasites may be too sparse to be seen easily in blood films, they grow well *in vitro* using a range of common media, including nutrient agar–blood mixtures, and also readily infect laboratory mice. A common and simple diagnostic procedure is to allow uninfected, laboratory-reared kissing bugs to feed on the patient and then to examine the bugs' faeces or gut contents three or four weeks later. If trypanosomes are present, it is clear that the patient was infected (but see *T. rangeli*, below). This technique is called xenodiagnosis.

Treatment

There is no really effective treatment for Chagas' disease. Two extremely toxic drugs are used, benznidazole and nifurtimox, but opinions are divided about their efficacy. There seems little doubt that they may be helpful if given early in the disease, though they are not necessarily so. Certainly they are not effective in the chronic phase. Different strains or zymodemes of the parasite may differ in their sensitivity to these drugs. The course of drug treatment is long.

Prevention and control

Well built, well maintained houses are unlikely to harbour bugs, and thus the best form of prevention is the improvement of living standards. Bed nets (mosquito nets) may help to prevent contact between bugs and sleepers, but only if they are carefully used and well maintained. Even then, in heavily infested houses, bugs crawling over the nets may subject the sleeper to a rain of infective faeces. Spraying inside houses with residual insecticide is effective but expensive.

T. cruzi infection is so widespread in some areas that infection via blood transfusion is a real risk. This can be prevented by adding gentian violet to the stored blood, but this has the unfortunate side effect of colouring the blood and, temporarily, the recipient, blue.

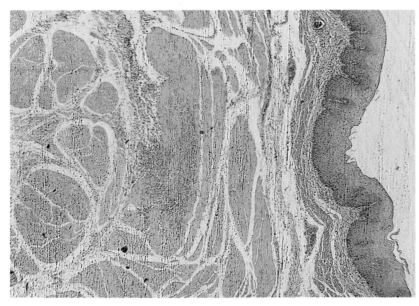

Fig. 1.54 Low powered photomicrograph of a section of human heart from a patient who died as a result of Chagas' disease; the characteristic infiltration of small round cells can be seen between the myofibrils. H & E stain.

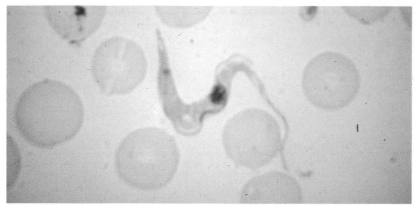

Fig. 1.55 Haematozoic trypomastigote of *T. rangeli* in blood of a dog. From a slide of the late Dr C A Hoare, courtesy of and © The Trustees of the Wellcome Trust 1988.

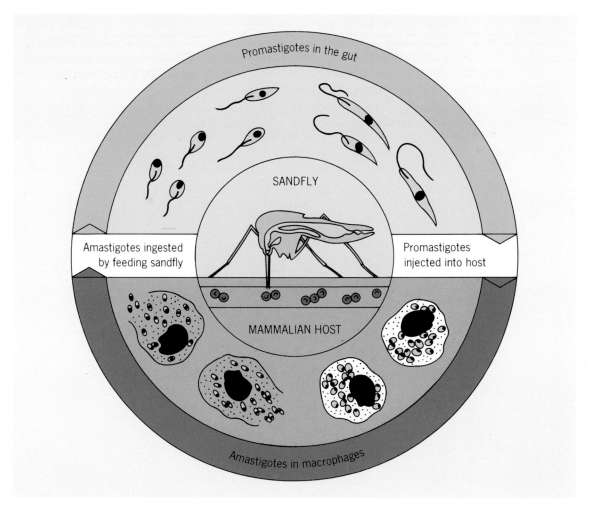

Fig. 1.56 The life cycle of *Leishmania*.

Causative organism	Disease
Trypanosoma rangeli	None

Trypanosoma rangeli occurs in the same areas of South America as *T. cruzi*, but is distributed more sporadically. It does infect man but causes no discernible sign or symptom of disease in human hosts. Even more unusually, it is pathogenic to its insect vectors, kissing bugs. It has some feral or wild reservoir hosts in common with *T. cruzi*.

The medical importance of *T. rangeli* is that if it occurs in blood films and kissing bugs, or cultures used for diagnosis, it may be mistaken for *T. cruzi*. Since the two species also share some antigens, serological testing may be unreliable. *T. rangeli* haematozoic trypomastigotes (Fig. 1.55) are longer (c.30μm) than those of *T. cruzi*, and the metacyclic forms which develop *in vitro* or in the vectors are also longer. Cross-reaction in serological tests can be minimized by careful choice and preparation of antigens and serial dilution of the test serum to an extent adequate to remove a weakly cross-reacting antigen. Confusion may be difficult to avoid if patients are infected with both species, but such confusion would not be clinically important.

LEISHMANIA

Leishmania species belong to the same family as *Trypanosoma* (the Trypanosomatidae), but they have a simpler life cycle (Fig. 1.56) existing in two forms only: amastigotes in their mammalian hosts, and promastigotes in their insect vectors. These vectors are small Diptera commonly known as sandflies (family Psychodidae, subfamily Phlebotominae, genus *Phlebotomus* and a few other closely related genera or subgenera). Only the females feed on blood.

Amastigotes are rounded forms, with virtually no flagellum. The amastigotes of most species of *Leishmania* are smaller than those of *T. cruzi*, measuring from 2 to 4μm in diameter (Fig. 1.57). Promastigotes are elongated, flagellate forms with the kinetoplast and flagellar basal body near the anterior end (Fig. 1.58). No sexual cycle is known, both forms reproducing by binary fission, though evidence suggestive of genetic exchange (as in *T. brucei*) is emerging.

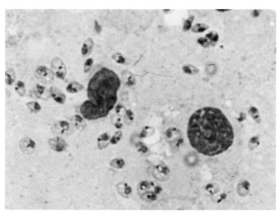

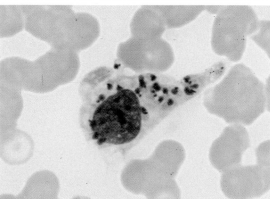

Fig. 1.57 Amastigotes of *L. donovani* in (upper) a Giemsa-stained smear of spleen from an experimentally infected mouse and (lower) within a bone marrow macrophage.

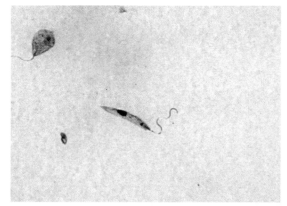

Fig. 1.58 Promastigote of *Leishmania* from a culture.

Causative organisms	Disease
Leishmania donovani	Visceral leishmaniasis
L. infantum, L. chagasi;	(including kala-azar)

In the 'Old World' (including Asia, Africa and southern Europe) there are two species, *L. donovani* and *L. infantum*, which some workers regard merely as subspecies. In the 'New World' (Central and South America), visceral leishmaniasis is caused by *L. chagasi* which, again, is regarded only as a subspecies by some authorities (Fig. 1.59).

Transmission and epidemiology

Transmission occurs when an infected sandfly bites a susceptible host. In the fly, the promastigotes develop first in the midgut and then migrate forward to the foregut and proboscis. There they become so numerous that some of them are swept down the proboscis when the insect feeds and ejects saliva into the puncture (the parasites do not invade the salivary glands of the fly). They then enter, or are ingested by, macrophages. They remain within phagosomes but, in some way which is not understood, resist digestion by the lysosomal enzymes and so survive to transform into amastigotes and divide. When a cell is full of amastigotes, it ruptures and the parasites emerge to re-enter other nearby macrophages. Some parasites enter macrophages which circulate in the blood (monocytes) and thus infect sandflies which feed subsequently.

In India, where classical kala-azar occurs, man is apparently the only mammalian host. In some parts of Africa *L. donovani* also infects dogs and some rodents which serve as reservoirs of human infection. Around the Mediterranean, *L. infantum* commonly infects dogs and, perhaps because of this, the disease more commonly affects children. The species (or subspecies) which has evolved to suit this rather different epidemiological situation is *L. infantum*. Dogs and wild canids are reservoir hosts of *L. chagasi* in the Americas.

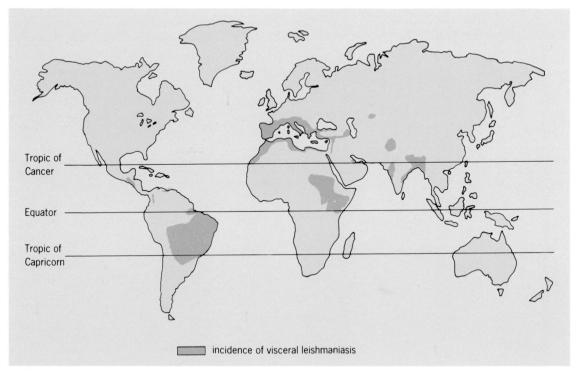

Fig. 1.59 The distribution of visceral leishmaniasis.

Clinical effects

As implied by the term 'visceral leishmaniasis', macrophages infected with *L. donovani*, *L. infantum* and *L. chagasi* congregate in the viscera, notably the spleen and liver, the fixed macrophages of the latter being the Kupffer cells, which line the blood sinuses (Fig. 1.60). These organs become hugely enlarged, and their functions are progressively impeded. A slow but progressive illness ensues, with bouts of irregularly recurring fever, which may be mild. Unless it is treated, the disease is invariably fatal.

Sometimes treatment of kala-azar is followed by a skin reaction, possibly allergic, in which nodules develop all over the body; these nodules contain parasitized macrophages. This condition is called post-kala-azar dermal leishmanoid.

Diagnosis

In endemic areas, a long-standing febrile illness with progressive enlargement of the liver and spleen but no other especially distinct sign is suggestive of visceral leishmaniasis. The only confirmatory diagnosis is demonstration of the parasites, either by microscopy (using Giemsa's or Leishman's stain) or, more sensitively, by growth (as promastigotes) in culture. Suitable culture media include the conventional nutrient agar–blood mixtures such as are used for *T. cruzi*. Material for microscopical examination or inoculation into culture may be obtained by aseptic puncture of sternal bone marrow or, more dangerously, from the enlarged spleen.

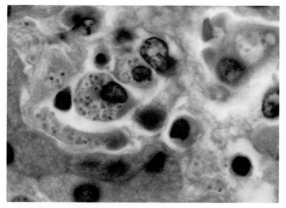

Fig. 1.60 Section of liver from a case of visceral leishmaniasis; amastigotes can be seen in the phagocytic Kupffer cells lining the blood sinuses. H & E stain.

Treatment

Visceral leishmaniasis is not easily treated. The preferred drugs are two compounds containing pentavalent antimony, sodium stibogluconate or meglumine antimonate; a prolonged course may be necessary. Pentamidine can be used if the antimonials are not effective.

Prevention and control

The only effective means of prevention are protection from sandfly bites and elimination of infected dogs in areas where they serve as reservoir hosts. Sandflies are so small that they can penetrate many mosquito nets.

Causative organisms	Diseases
Leishmania aethiopica *L. major*, *L. tropica*	Old World cutaneous leishmaniasis (*L. aethiopica* may cause disseminated cutaneous leishmaniasis (DCL))
L. mexicana complex, *L. braziliensis* complex	New World cutaneous leishmaniasis (*L. braziliensis* may also cause mucocutaneous leishmaniasis or *espundia*; *L. mexicana* may cause DCL)
L. peruviana	Peruvian cutaneous leishmaniasis or *uta*

Transmission and epidemiology

Transmission of these species is by the bite of an infected sandfly. Development in the fly, and in macrophages of the mammalian host, is similar to that described above (although the site in the body where the infected cells localize is different: see below).

L. mexicana infection is usually acquired away from human habitation, in the forest, as the commoner reservoir hosts are wild rodents. The same is true of *L. braziliensis*, the reservoirs of which are mainly rodents and sloths. *L. peruviana* is unusual: it occurs in the cold highlands of Peru only, and the reservoirs are dogs. These three species occur only in the Americas: *L. braziliensis* is less restricted geographically than *L. peruviana*, being found throughout Central and South America; *L. mexicana* is the most widespread, occurring also in southern USA (Texas) and (as its name implies) Mexico (Fig. 1.61).

In the 'Old World', *L. major* exists in Asia and Africa; gerbils and other rodents are reservoir hosts. *L. aethiopica* has been recorded from East and Northeast Africa only; the hyrax is a reservoir host. *L. tropica* exists around the Mediterranean basin (southern Europe and north Africa) and eastwards through Asia to India; dogs may act as reservoir hosts in some areas but this is uncertain.

Clinical effects

All these organisms are essentially confined to the skin of their mammalian hosts, perhaps because they are more sensitive to high temperatures than *L.* *donovani* and related 'visceral' species. The extent of the disease they cause may vary widely and many subspecies are recognized clinically and on other grounds such as isoenzyme electrophoresis.

L. tropica, *L. major* and *L. mexicana* cause only one or a few lesions at the site of the infected bite (Fig. 1.62). They do not spread to other sites, and considerable immunity usually follows infection. *L. peruviana* behaves similarly. *L. aethopica* is normally restricted to a single lesion but under certain conditions, perhaps when the host is immunologically compromised, it may spread widely throughout the skin producing a seriously disfiguring condition, disseminated cutaneous leishmaniasis (DCL) (Fig. 1.63); this is not unlike leprosy in appearance and is very difficult to cure. Two other species related to *L. mexicana*, *L. amazonensis* and *L. pifanoi*, may also give rise to DCL.

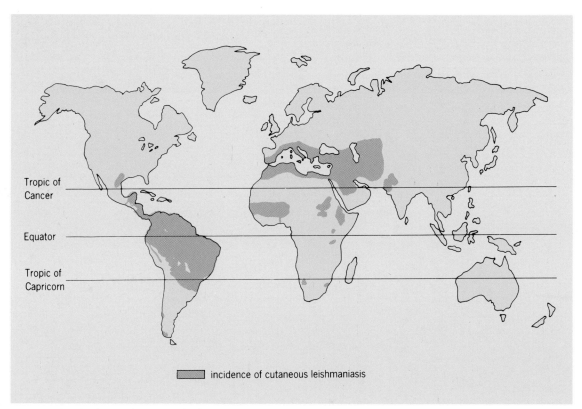

Fig. 1.61 The distribution of cutaneous leishmaniasis.

L. braziliensis is often restricted to single skin lesions, but may sometimes spread to the muco-cutaneous junction in the pharynx and cause complete breakdown of the palate and roof of the mouth, and the nose. This is known as mucocutaneous leishmaniasis or *espundia*.

Sections of infected skin in all these conditions reveal parasitized macrophages and a surrounding inflammatory reaction involving infiltration of large numbers of lymphocytic cells (Fig. 1.64).

Diagnosis

Cutaneous leishmaniasis is diagnosed by microscopic examination or culture. To obtain suitable material for examination, it is usual to puncture the margin of a lesion with a hypodermic needle (using aseptic procedure), attached to a syringe which may contain a very small amount of normal saline. The aspirate contained in the needle is then expelled on to a microscope slide or into a tube of culture medium. The periphery, rather than the centre, of a lesion is used because the centre is often filled with tissue debris and dead material with no living parasites present.

Treatment

Sodium stibogluconate and meglumine antimonate are used to treat cutaneous leishmaniasis. If the

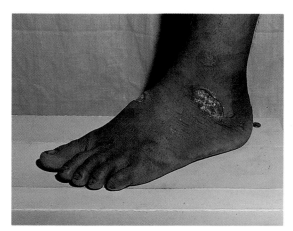

Fig. 1.62 Skin lesion caused by *L. mexicana*. Courtesy of Dr J J Shaw.

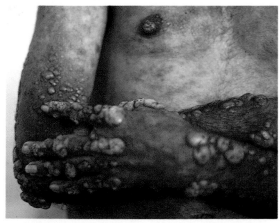

Fig. 1.63 Disseminated cutaneous leishmaniasis due to *L. amazonensis*. Courtesy of Dr J J Shaw.

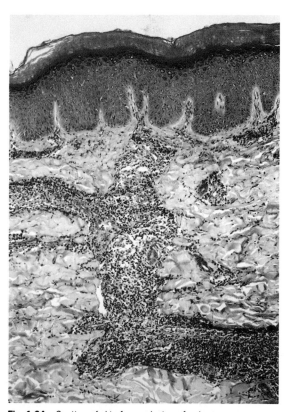

Fig. 1.64 Section of skin from a lesion of cutaneous leishmaniasis (*L. tropica*), showing parasitized macrophages and lymphocytic infiltration in the dermis. H & E stain. Courtesy of Dr J J Shaw.

condition fails to respond, pentamidine or amphotericin B can be tried.

If the patient has uncomplicated cutaneous leishmaniasis, with only a single skin lesion, treatment is usually unnecessary as the condition will heal spontaneously and probably leave the patient with some immunity to reinfection. If, however, there is a possibility of mucocutaneous leishmaniasis or DCL developing, treatment should certainly be given.

Prevention and control

The only sure way to prevent infection is by avoiding the bite of infected sandflies, which is almost impossible for persons living or working in forests and other areas where the infection is endemic. Protective clothing, insect repellants and insecticidal sprays inside huts and houses may help.

PARASITES OF THE GASTROINTESTINAL AND UROGENITAL SYSTEMS

Causative organism	Disease
Giardia lamblia	Giardiasis (lambliasis)

Transmission and epidemiology

Giardia has a worldwide distribution. The trophozoites (Fig. 1.65) have two nuclei, four pairs of flagella and one or two curved median bodies of unknown function, which are sometimes incorrectly called parabasal bodies. The trophozoites, measuring 10–20μm long, 5–10μm broad and 2–4μm thick, multiply by binary fission, and no sexual phase is known.

The infective stage of *G. lamblia* is a resistant cyst (Fig. 1.66). The oval cysts measuring 6–10μm × 8–14μm are passed out in the faeces and ingested in contaminated water and food. Cysts are often waterborne, either by inadequately treated municipal water supplies or in contaminated rivers or streams. Infection from river water has occurred among campers in the USA where beavers are thought to be reservoir hosts supplying the cysts. Monkeys and pigs can also be infected, and infected pigs may sometimes be a source of human infection.

Clinical effects

Giardia inhabits the duodenum and upper ileum. The trophozoites browse on the mucosal surface, to which they are attached by an oval, ventral anterior disc, or sucker (Fig. 1.67). If present in large numbers they damage the mucosa and cause atrophy of the villi, but they do not penetrate the surface.

Heavy infections produce severe, bloodless diarrhoea, especially in young children. If the parasites swim up the bile duct to the gall bladder, nausea, vomiting and jaundice may ensue. Villous atrophy may interfere with the absorption of food, especially fats and fat-soluble vitamins; consequently the diarrhoeic faeces may be fatty (steatorrhoea). There may be epigastric pain.

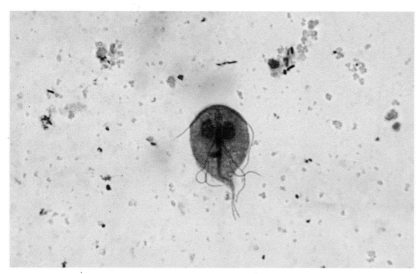

Fig. 1.65 Trophozoite of *Giardia lamblia*. The organism (seen here in face view) is shaped like a longitudinally bisected pear. The rim of the ventral attachment disc can be seen around the broader, anterior region. Giemṣa's stain.

Diagnosis

The diagnosis can be confirmed only by identifying cysts during microscopical examination of faecal specimens. Cysts are usually numerous and easily recognized by their shape, number of nuclei and confused jumble of flagella, even in unstained specimens. They may be more difficult to find if, as sometimes happens, treatment has cleared the intestinal infection but some parasites remain in the biliary system.

Treatment

Metronidazole, tinidazole or other 5-nitroimidazole compounds usually kill parasites in the intestine, but any in the gall bladder or bile duct may evade destruction and subsequently reinvade the intestine to produce clinical relapse. If this occurs, repeated courses of therapy at higher doses may be required.

Prevention and control

Suspect water should be boiled or adequately filtered to remove the infective cysts before drinking.

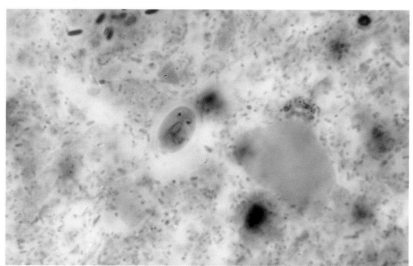

Fig. 1.66 An oval cyst of *G. lamblia* containing four nuclei (only two are clearly visible), the remnants of the median bodies and flagella, and the rim of the attachment disc. Iron haematoxylin stain.

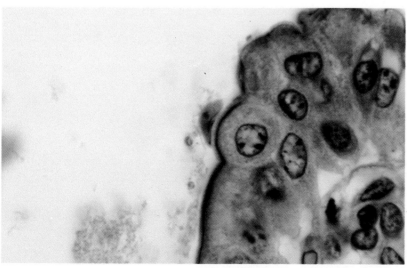

Fig. 1.67 *G. lamblia* trophozoite lying on the mucosal surface of the small intestine. Iron haematoxylin stain.

Chemical purification with chlorine or iodine is less reliable. In endemic areas, raw vegetables should be washed in boiled water or, preferably, avoided.

Epidemics arising from piped water supplies can be controlled by repairing the fault in the system which allowed the cysts to enter the supply.

Causative organism	Disease
Trichomonas vaginalis	Trichomonas vaginitis or trichomonas urethritis

Transmission and epidemiology
The trophozoites of *Trichomonas*, measuring 14–17μm × 5–15μm have a single nucleus, four anterior flagella and a single lateral flagellum attached to the pellicle to form an undulating membrane (Fig. 1.68). The inner margin of this membrane is supported by a filament. There is also a central skeletal rod or axostyle.

Trichomonas vaginalis (Fig. 1.69) inhabits the vagina of women and the urethra (and sometimes prostate) of men; it multiplies by binary fission (Fig. 1.70). It is transmitted during sexual intercourse, and no encysted stage is known. Up to 40 per cent of women have been reported in some random surveys to be infected, and the organism has been found in up to 70 per cent of women with vaginitis.

Clinical effects
In men, *T. vaginalis* is rarely pathogenic, though it may produce mild urethritis or prostatitis.

In women, it is often non-pathogenic, but heavy infections (associated with a reduction in the acidity of vaginal secretions from pH 4–4.5 to around pH 5) may cause mild to severe vaginitis, with copious foul-smelling discharge.

Diagnosis
Clinical suspicion may be confirmed by finding trophozoites in Giemsa-stained smears made from swabs of the vaginal discharge or, in difficult cases, by cultivation of the swab plus discharge at 37°C in various culture media (for example, Lowe's, a nutrient broth plus horse serum and antibiotics).

Treatment
5-Nitroimidazoles (for example, metronidazole, tinidazole) are usually used, given orally. Radical cure may be difficult due to the problem of obtaining an adequate drug concentration in the vagina. If an infected woman has a regular sexual partner, he must be treated also, or the woman will be reinfected.

Prevention and control
Sexual abstinence or regular use of condoms will prevent infection but the disease produced (if any) may not be considered severe enough to justify such

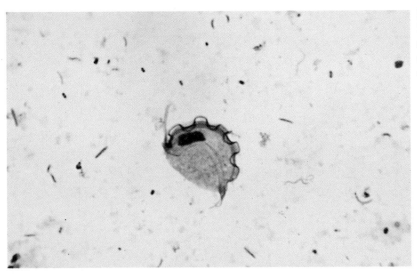

Fig. 1.68 Trophozoite of *Trichomonas muris*. In this specimen the lateral flagellum extends just beyond the posterior end of the organism. Giemsa's stain.

action. Promiscuity clearly increases the risk of infection; regular sexual partners can be treated, if necessary, to abolish the source of infection.

NON-PATHOGENIC FLAGELLATES

Other flagellates, which are harmless commensals, may inhabit the gastrointestinal tract of man. Their only medical significance is the possibility of their confusion with *Giardia lamblia*. *Trichomonas tenax* lives in the mouth. *Dientamoeba fragilis* used to be classified as an amoeba but is now thought to be an aberrant flagellate; although binucleate, it has no flagella or median bodies. *T. tenax* and *D. fragilis* do not produce cysts.

Chilomastix mesnili, *Enteromonas hominis*, *Retortamonas intestinalis* and *Trichomonas* (or *Pentatrichomonas*) *hominis* can be distinguished from *G. lamblia* in the trophozoite stage. They have only one nucleus and five or fewer flagella; their cysts can be distinguished from those of *G. lamblia* by the absence of remnants of flagella, median bodies and the rim of the adhesive disc.

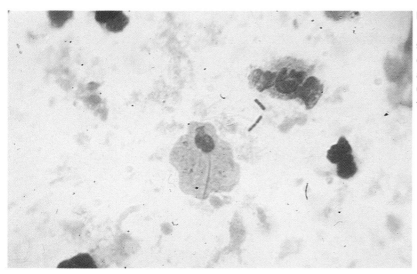

Fig. 1.69 Trophozoite of *T. vaginalis* in a smear of vaginal secretion; the lateral flagellum extends typically about half-way along the cell. Giemsa's stain. Courtesy and © The Trustees of the Wellcome Trust 1988.

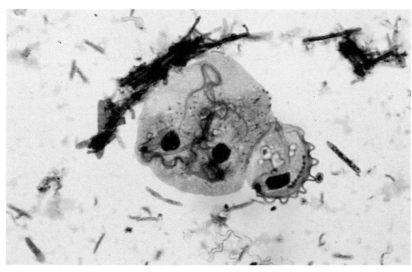

Fig. 1.70 Two trophozoites of *Trichomonas* sp.; that on the left is dividing (note the two nuclei). Giemsa's stain.

AMOEBAE OF THE GASTROINTESTINAL TRACT

Causative organism	Disease
Entamoeba histolytica	Amoebic dysentery, amoebiasis

Transmission and epidemiology

Entamoeba histolytica inhabits the lumen of the large intestine of man and other primates, dogs, cats, pigs and rodents; it may invade the mucosa and other viscera. Man is the main, and probably the only, natural host. The disease, though not the organism itself, seems to occur only in the tropics and sub-tropics. Reports of *E. histolytica* infections from temperate regions are probably often misidentifications of *E. hartmanni* (see p.49), though some may refer to non-pathogenic 'strains' of *E. histolytica*

(p.47); also, persons who are infected in warmer countries may travel to temperate regions and develop the clinical disease there.

The trophozoite (Fig. 1.71), irregular in shape and measuring from 10–40μm in diameter, reproduces by binary fission. No sexual phase is known but recent, indirect evidence suggests the possibility of some kind of genetic exchange. The transmission stage is a resistant cyst, typically spherical and measuring from 9.5–15.5μm in diameter (Fig. 1.72), excreted in the faeces and ingested with contaminated food and water. Human infections probably derive directly from other infected humans; although dogs, cats and rats may occasionally be sources of infection, it is likely that they are more often infected from humans. Most infected people are asymptomatic cyst-passers who may act as reservoir hosts, especially if they are food-handlers by profession.

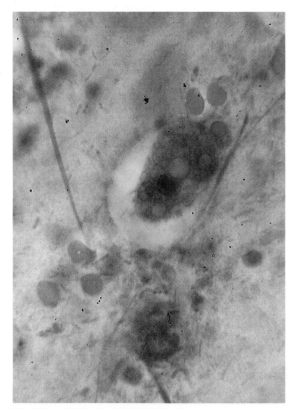

Fig. 1.71 *Entamoeba histolytica*: trophozoite containing ingested erythrocyte and a characteristic entamoeba-type nucleus resembling a wheel, with a peripheral stained rim and a small central karyosome. H & E stain.

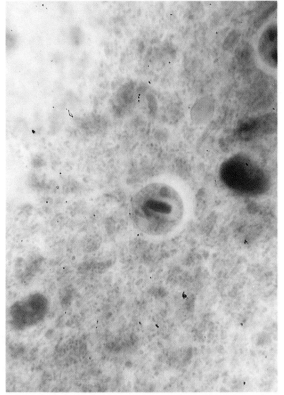

Fig. 1.72 Cyst of *E. histolytica*. Only one of the four nuclei is visible but a characteristically shaped broad chromatoid bar, with rounded ends, can be seen; it is a semi-crystalline aggregation of ribosomes. H & E stain.

Coprophagous insects may help to disseminate the infection to a small extent, by mechanical carriage of cysts on their feet from faeces to food.

Clinical effects

Most human infections are harmless, the amoebae merely living in the gut lumen as commensals. Occasionally, for reasons not yet fully understood (but probably programmed into the genome of particular 'strains'), the trophozoites penetrate the intestinal mucosa and multiply in the submucosa (Fig. 1.73), forming flask-shaped ulcers. This process may result in diarrhoea or acute dysentery; the stools usually contain amoebic trophozoites as well as blood and mucus.

From these ulcers, the amoebae may enter blood vessels and be carried to other organs, most commonly the liver, via the hepatic portal system (Fig. 1.74). Here they may settle and multiply to form amoebic 'abscesses' (not strictly abscesses as they are bacteriologically sterile), which may be several centimetres in diameter. Rarely, these lesions occur in lung, skin or even brain.

Submucosal ulcers, and 'abscesses' in the liver, may (rarely) rupture into the peritoneum and cause acute peritonitis, which can be fatal. Cysts are never formed in the tissues.

Diagnosis

Confirmatory diagnosis depends on identifying the amoebae (see chapter 4). This can be done by direct microscopy of faecal preparations but, especially in asymptomatic infections, the parasites may be scanty. In such cases, faeces can be cultured in suitable media, so that the parasites increase in number to an easily detectable level. Serological

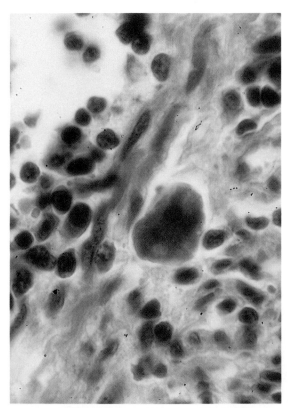

Fig. 1.73 Section of part of an amoebic ulcer, showing a trophozoite of *E. histolytica* in the submucosa. H & E stain.

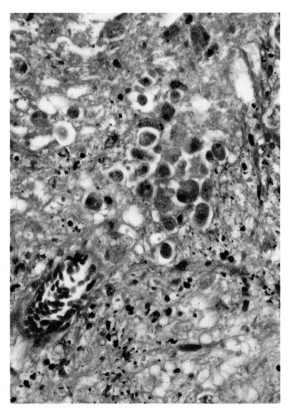

Fig. 1.74 Trophozoites of *E. histolytica* in a liver 'abscess'. H & E stain (low power).

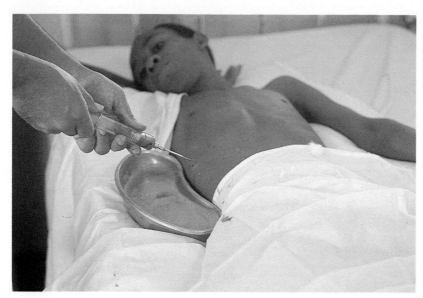

Fig. 1.75 Patient having pus (named 'anchovy-sauce' pus from the characteristic colour) drained from an amoebic liver abscess.

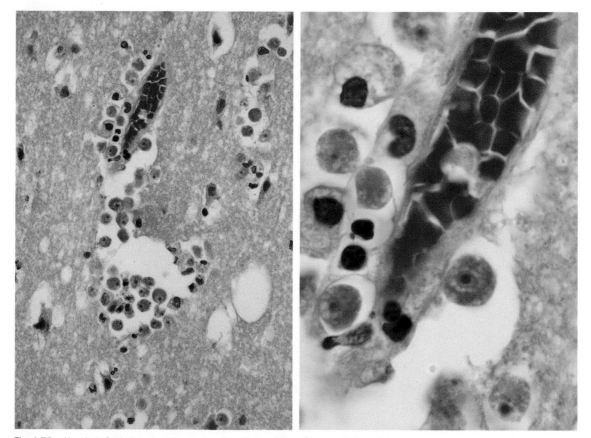

Fig. 1.76 *Naegleria fowleri* trophozoites in a post-mortem section of human brain. Left: low-power photomicrograph. Right: high-power photomicrograph.

techniques are useful to detect possible tissue invasion, but are rarely positive in lumen-only infections and so are no help in detecting potentially infectious cyst-passers.

Treatment

Radical cure is not always easy to attain. Older drugs still in use include emetine and its less-toxic derivative, dehydroemetine, both given intramuscularly. Orally administered 5-nitroimidazoles (metronidazole and tinidazole) are now commonly used, sometimes with tetracycline. Oral chloroquine (an antimalarial drug) kills amoebae in liver lesions but not elsewhere. Large 'abscesses' may require surgical drainage (Fig. 1.75).

Prevention and control

The prevalence of asymptomatic infections means that food-handlers in endemic areas should, ideally, be screened by faecal examination and, if infected, treated. Food should be protected from cockroaches and flies, and piped water supplies should be well maintained to avoid contamination.

NON-PATHOGENIC AMOEBAE

Several amoebae dwell harmlessly in the human intestine and are possible causes of misdiagnosis. These species are:

- *Entamoeba coli*, cysts larger than *E. histolytica*, with eight nuclei when mature

- *Entamoeba hartmanni*, cysts smaller than those of *E. histolytica* but with four nuclei and chromatoid bars of *E. histolytica* type

- *Endolimax nana*, small oval cyst with no chromatoid bars and four nuclei, not of *Entamoeba* type

- *Iodamoeba buetschlii*, uninucleate cyst, commonly with large vacuole containing glycogen which stains dark brown with iodine

- *Entamoeba gingivalis* lives as a harmless commensal in the human mouth; it does not encyst.

A rather enigmatic organism, quite often seen in faecal preparations, is *Blastocystis hominis*. This parasite was regarded as a yeast-like fungus, and still is by many workers, but there is some evidence that it may be a protozoon, possibly an amoeba. Its presence in the gut is not associated with any clinical condition but, again, some workers believe that it may, occasionally, be associated with, if not cause, a diarrhoeic syndrome. The infection is said to respond to metronidazole treatment. It is just possible that *B. hominis* may become clinically relevant in immunocompromised persons in future.

FACULTATIVELY PARASITIC AMOEBAE

Causative organism	Disease
Naegleria fowleri	Primary amoebic
Naegleria australiensis	meningoencephalitis (PAM)
Acanthamoeba culbertsoni	Granulomatous amoebic encephalitis (GAE)

Transmission and epidemiology

These amoebae are normally free-living. *Naegleria* spp. have flagellate, amoeboid and encysted stages in their life cycles, the flagellate in water and the latter two in soil or mud at the bottom of ponds. *Acanthamoeba* has no flagellate stage; the amoebae (trophozoites and encysted forms) live in soil. Reported human infections due to *Naegleria* are few in number (below 200) but usually fatal in outcome. The parasites are restricted to relatively warm water, usually in the tropics or subtropics, though one fatal infection was acquired from warm spa water at Bath, UK; heated swimming pools are another possible source of infection. Infection apparently occurs when the amoeboid stage is forced up the nose of persons swimming in, or jumping into, water containing the parasites. Penetrating the mucous membrane at the back of the nose, the amoebae migrate up the olfactory nerve to the brain (Fig. 1.76).

Naegleria australiensis infects mice experimentally in a similar way and is therefore suspected of being able to infect man.

Acanthamoeba culbertsoni has been found in the brain of a few (fewer than 50) human patients, most of whom have been immunodeficient in some way, and in the throats of infants (and a few older persons) in the USA. It seems likely that the amoeba enters the mouth of crawling children in soil or dust (possibly encysted) and sometimes becomes established, producing more or less asymptomatic infections. In immunodeficient individuals, it may then penetrate the mucosa and reach the brain, causing granulomatous amoebic encephalitis. It is possible that the prevalence of this type of infection will increase with the advent of AIDS. Both primary amoebic meningo-encephalitis and granulomatous amoebic encephalitis are widely distributed around the world.

Clinical effects

Naegleria produces signs and symptoms typical of acute meningitis: headache, stiff neck, vomiting and fever, followed in a few days by drowsiness and coma. Microscopically, the picture is of diffuse, fulminating meningitis with infiltration of the meninges, predominantly by polymorphonuclear leucocytes. *N. fowleri* does not encyst in tissue lesions.

A. culbertsoni produces a less acute illness; mental confusion, dizziness, drowsiness and other signs may appear slowly, followed by coma. Microscopically, typical granulomas with multinucleate giant cells are seen; *A. culbertsoni* does encyst in lesions, so cysts may be seen as well as trophozoites.

Diagnosis

Infections of the throat by *A. culbertsoni* can be diagnosed by examining or culturing mucus from swabs. Diagnoses of PAM and GAE have usually been made post mortem. However, a presumptive diagnosis is possible in patients with acute encephalitis, not of bacterial aetiology, with a recent history of swimming in warm, muddy water. Examination of the cerebrospinal fluid may reveal parasites and is the only means of establishing diagnosis before death. Material can be examined by direct microscopy or after cultivation *in vitro*.

Treatment

The rapidity of PAM and the difficulty of diagnosing this and GAE before death make treatment difficult. Some successes have been claimed for the use of amphotericin B plus tetracycline, or rifampicin plus miconazole, provided treatment can be started sufficiently early.

Prevention and control

Infection can be prevented only by avoiding swimming in warm, muddy water. The only method of control is to identify potentially manageable possible

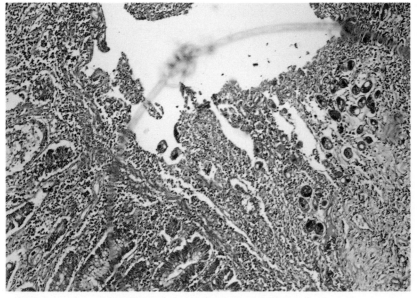

Fig. 1.77 Trophozoites of *B. coli* in an ulcer within the submucosa, low power micrograph.

sources of infection, such as inadequately maintained swimming baths, clean them using hypochlorite solution or other suitable disinfectants, and prevent reinfection of the water by adequate filtration and chemical treatment (such as adequate chlorination).

CILIATES

Causative organism	Disease
Balantidium coli	Balantidial dysentery; balantidiasis

Transmission and epidemiology

Balantidium coli is the only ciliate parasite which infects man. Its natural host is the pig, in which asymptomatic infections of the lumen of the large intestine are common throughout the world. The parasite may be pathogenic to pigs if damage to the intestinal mucosa by some other cause, for example, *Salmonella* infection, allows it to penetrate to the submucosa. *B. coli* exists as a large, free-swimming ciliate and as an encysted form excreted in the faeces and forming the transmissive stage. The tropho-zoites, measuring $60–70\mu$m $\times$ $40–60\mu$m, reproduce both asexually (by transverse fission) and sexually by conjugation. All ciliates possess two nuclei; a large somatic, polyploid macronucleus and a small, haploid micronucleus active only during sexual reproduction.

Most (if not all) human infections are acquired by the accidental ingestion of cysts on food (for example, uncooked vegetables) contaminated with pig faeces. Man-to-man transmission, though theoretically possible, has never been demonstrated conclusively. Human infections are rare and usually occur in farm workers and other rural dwellers.

Clinical effects

Clinically, balantidial dysentery is indistinguishable from amoebic dysentery. Similar flask-shaped ulcers are found in the submucosa of the large intestine (Figs 1.77 and 1.78) and similar bloody dysentery results. *B. coli* has not been recorded from any other viscera, and neither have asymptomatic infections of the bowel lumen been reported from man; it would not, however, be surprising if the latter occurred.

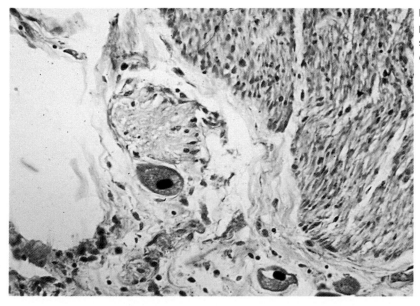

Fig. 1.78 Higher powered photomicrograph of *B. coli* in submucosa, showing the characteristic large macronucleus.

Diagnosis

Balantidiasis is fairly easily diagnosed by finding the large, spherical cysts (50–60μm in diameter) by microscopical examination of faecal preparations.

Treatment

As with *Entamoeba histolytica*, metronidazole or other 5-nitroimidazoles are commonly used.

Prevention and control

Food contaminated by pig faeces should be avoided.

CRYPTOSPORIDIUM

Causative organism	Disease
Cryptosporidium muris	Cryptosporidiosis

Transmission and epidemiology

Cryptosporidium muris is an apicomplexan parasite which, until recently, was not known to infect man but was thought to be restricted to a range of other mammals including rodents and many domestic animals. In spite of minor differences between strains

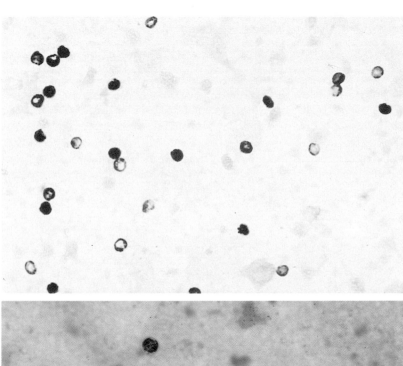

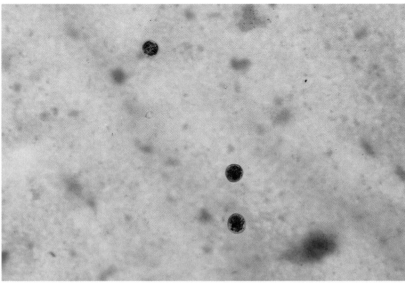

Fig. 1.79 *Cryptosporidium* oocysts in unconcentrated faecal specimens, low and high power light micrographs; modified acid-fast stain. Courtesy of Dr S Tzipori.

infecting these various hosts, all are thought to belong to the same species. Human infection was first reported in 1976; since then the organism has been reported in from 1 to 4 per cent of patients with diarrhoea in developed countries and in up to 16 per cent in less developed countries. It is most common in children; most immunocompetent adults seem to be immune, but in those who are immunodeficient, for any reason, intense infections may develop.

C. muris needs only a single host in its life cycle. Transmission is by means of a resistant oocyst, passed out in the faeces and ingested with contaminated food or water. Four sporozoites are liberated from the oocyst. They enter cells of the microvillous border of the small intestine, remaining very superficial in the cell but beneath its plasmalemma, within a membrane-bound parasitophorous vacuole. Here they undergo merogony and, finally, gametogony, to give rise to sexual individuals (gametocytes) which develop into gametes; fusion of the latter results in a diploid zygote which encysts to form the infective oocyst. The life cycle is essentially similar to that of *Plasmodium* (pp. 4–8), although no second vector host is involved.

Some thin-walled oocysts apparently hatch within the intestine of the same host, thereby building up the infection to a very high level if the host is unable to control it immunologically. Other oocysts are excreted and recommence development only when swallowed by another, susceptible, host.

It is thought that rodents and domestic animals may act as a source of human infection, but infections of people are thought usually to result from person to person transmission.

Clinical effects

Infection with *C. muris* causes diarrhoea; a few asymptomatic infections have been reported, but these seem to be rare, or perhaps overlooked. In immunocompetent people, the diarrhoea is rarely severe and usually self-limiting, but in those who are immunodeficient it can be severe, intractable, and even life-threatening. The diarrhoea results from non-inflammatory gastroenteritis, neither blood nor pus being present in the stool. Stool volumes of up to 25 litres per day have been recorded. Vomiting sometimes occurs, and this may account for the

relatively rare complication of pulmonary cryptosporidiosis.

Diagnosis

Diagnosis depends on identification of the oocysts in faeces. As the oocysts are very small (4–6μm in diameter), this is not easy. Concentration by flotation techniques (chapter 4) followed by staining with acid-fast stains (such as Ziehl–Neelsen) make the oocysts easier to find (Fig. 1.79). Serological tests can be used to detect serum antibodies, but these remain positive for at least several months after initial infection and so are not of much use in the diagnosis of acute cryptosporidiosis.

Treatment

This is unnecessary in immunocompetent persons. In those who are not immunocompetent, treatment so far has been almost uniformly unsuccessful. The only chemotherapy which has shown any promise is administration of spiramycin, 1–3g daily for 2–4 weeks, and this is not always effective. One agammaglobulinaemic child with cryptosporidiosis appeared to respond favourably to oral administration of hyperimmune bovine colostrum, so perhaps this treatment should be further investigated.

Prevention and control

As with all intestinal infections, this can be prevented only by avoiding the ingestion of infective stages by hygienic precautions in the preparation of uncooked food, and protection of such food from contamination with oocysts from the faeces of infected rodents and other reservoir hosts. Particular care should be taken by those involved in the care of infected persons, or by those known to be immunoincompetent.

MICROSPORIDA

Causative organisms	Disease
Enterocytozoon bieneusi	Microsporidiasis
Encephalitozoon cuniculi	
Nosema connori	
?Pleistophora sp.	

Transmission and pathology

Enterocytozoon bieneusi was first described in 1985,

and has now been reported from at least eight patients with AIDS; it inhabits mucosal cells of the small intestine (Fig. 1.80). *Encephalitozoon cuniculi* (Fig. 1.81) has long been known as a common, worldwide parasite of rodents, rabbits and carnivores; there are a few recorded infections in monkeys.

Two cases of human infection with *E. cuniculi* have been reported, one in Japan (1959) and one in Sweden (1984); both these infections were self-limiting. *Nosema connori* was described from an immunodeficient human infant in 1974; other species of *Nosema* are common parasites of arthropods throughout the world.

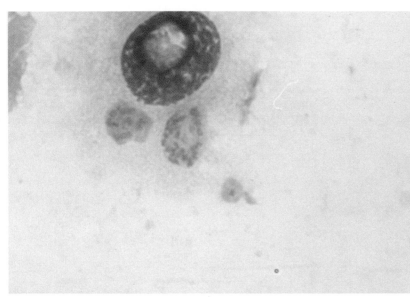

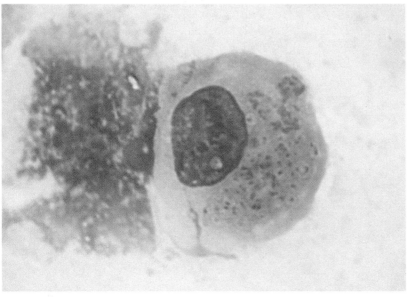

Fig. 1.80 *Enterocytozoon bieneusi* within cells from a human small intestine biopsy. Lower: spores have been formed in this cell. Giemsa's stain. Courtesy of Prof. E U Canning.

There have been two reports of unidentified Microsporida infecting human corneas. Another report, from an immunodeficient man in the USA (1985), was ascribed to *Pleistophora*, species of which normally infect fish or amphibians. It is perhaps significant that most of the human infections have been either in persons known to be immunodeficient, or in immunologically privileged sites (corneas) of presumably immunocompetent individuals.

Microsporida are transmitted as small spores, usually about $5 \times 2\mu$m. After being swallowed, the spore ejects a hollow, tubular polar filament which

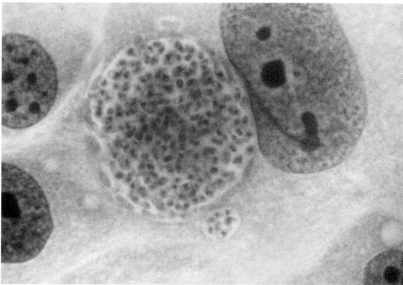

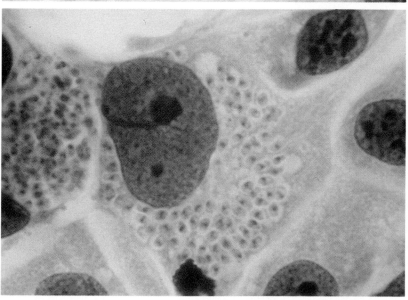

Fig. 1.81 *Encephalitozoon cuniculi* growing in cultured Madin–Derby canine kidney (MDCK) cells; intracellular spores have been formed in the cell shown below. Giemsa's stain. Courtesy of Prof. E U Canning.

penetrates the host cell and through which the sporo-plasm (infective contents of the spore) migrates into the host cell cytoplasm (Fig. 1.82). Here cycles of multiple fission (merogony and sporogony) occur, resulting in the production of more spores. In human corneal infection, it is possible that the infection of the eye occurred directly and not by ingestion of spores. Apart from *E. bieneusi*, the human infections presumably represent 'opportunistic' infection by species normally parasitizing other host species; whether this is also true of *E. bieneusi* is not yet clear.

Serological surveys using *E. cuniculi* antigen have revealed a surprisingly high prevalence of positive reactions among persons with tropical diseases. In Sweden, a survey of persons returning from tropical countries found 12 per cent to be positive for serum antibodies to *E. cuniculi*, up to 38 per cent in persons with malaria and over 40 per cent in those with tuberculosis. This raises several questions:

● do these cases represent subclinical infection or passive exposure to antigen?

● is the association with other infections due to an immunosuppressive effect of the concurrent disease?

● does it represent a common incidence of infection in tropical countries?

● could the positive reactions be due to cross–reacting antibodies arising from subclinical infection with *E. bieneusi*?

These questions cannot yet be answered, but it seems likely that, with the increasing prevalence of AIDS, human infections with Microsporida will become increasingly common, or at least increasingly recognized as clinically significant.

Clinical effects

The two human beings infected with *E. cuniculi* had severe but self-limiting neurological disease; spores were found in the cerebrospinal fluid of one patient, and in the urine of both. *N. connori* produced a disseminated, fatal infection in the immunodeficient infant, spores being found in most viscera, including kidney tubules and lungs; the child was also infected with *Pneumocystis carinii*. The *Pleistophora* infection was restricted to the muscle cells and resulted in severe febrile myositis with lymphadenopathy. Infection with *E. bieneusi* is associated with severe intractable diarrhoea.

Diagnosis

A rise in specific antibody titre between successive serological tests suggests active infection but this can be confirmed only by finding spores. In the three known cases, these were found in the cerebrospinal fluid and urine in one case, in the cornea in the second, and were disseminated in many organs in the third.

Treatment

Unknown as yet.

Prevention and control

It is impossible to suggest means of prevention and control until the source of the rare human infections is known. Hygienic disposal of fomites and excreta of any known human cases would be wise to prevent onward transmission, and perhaps isolation of the patient and adequate protection of those nursing him or her.

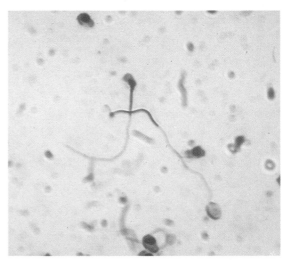

Fig. 1.82 Spore of the microsporan genus *Unikaryon* showing extruded polar filament , down which the darkly stained sporoplasm is passing. Courtesy of Prof. E U Canning.

2. HELMINTHS

TREMATODES

Adult trematodes, often known as flukes, may inhabit the intestinal tract, bile ducts, lungs or blood of man.

Trematodes are members of the phylum Platyhelminthes which also includes the cestodes or tapeworms. They are characteristically flat, leaf-like, hermaphroditic organisms (Fig. 2.1); except for the schistosomes which have a boat-shaped male and a cylindrical female. All have complicated life cycles with an alternating sexual cycle in the final host and an asexual multiplicative cycle in a gastropod snail intermediate host. In addition, many trematodes have a second intermediate host (*see* Fig. 2.2).

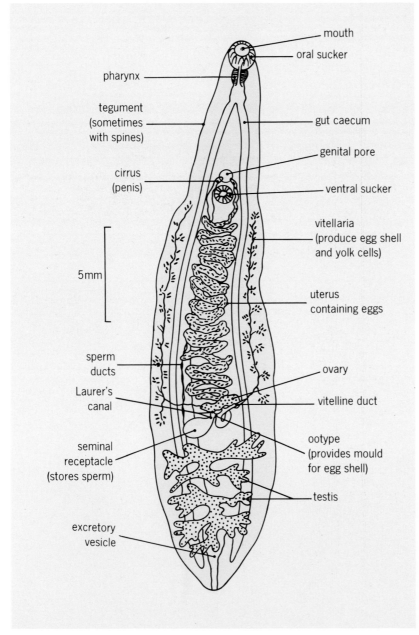

Fig. 2.1 Diagram of adult *Clonorchis sinensis* showing typical trematode features.

mouth

oral sucker

pharynx

tegument (sometimes with spines)

gut caecum

genital pore

cirrus (penis)

ventral sucker

vitellaria (produce egg shell and yolk cells)

5mm

uterus containing eggs

sperm ducts

ovary

Laurer's canal

vitelline duct

seminal receptacle (stores sperm)

ootype (provides mould for egg shell)

testis

excretory vesicle

Name of trematode	Habitat and genus of snail intermediate host	Mode of infection of man	Definitive hosts
Schistosoma japonicum	Banks of rivers and rice paddies (*Oncomelania*)	Active penetration of skin by cercariae	Man, Dog, Cattle, Rat
S. mansoni	Slow flowing rivers, canals and lakes (*Biomphalaria*)	Active penetration of skin by cercariae	Man, Rodents, (Baboon)
S. haematobium & *S. intercalatum*	Ponds and margins of lakes (*Bulinus*)	Active penetration of skin by cercariae	Man
Clonorchis sinensis	Slow flowing streams (*Bulinus*, *Parafossarulus*)	Cercariae encyst as metacercariae in freshwater fish	Man, Carnivores
Opisthorchis viverrini	Slow flowing streams (*Bithynia*)	Cercariae encyst as metacercariae in freshwater fish	Civet cat, Man
O. felineus	Slow flowing streams (*Bithynia*)	Cercariae encyst as metacercariae in freshwater fish	(Man) Cat
Paragonimus westermani	Fast flowing mountain streams (*Semisulcospira*, *Thiara*, *Oncomelania*)	Cercariae encyst as metacercariae in crabs and crayfish	Man, Carnivores
Paragonimus species	Fast flowing mountain streams (Various)	Cercariae encyst as metacercariae in crabs and crayfish	Carnivores (Man)
Fasciola hepatica	Damp pastures (*Lymnaea*)	Cercariae encyst as metacercariae on herbage	Sheep, Cattle (Man)
F. gigantica	Ponds (*Lymnaea*)	Cercariae encyst as metacercariae on herbage	Cattle (Man?)
Fasciolopsis buski	Ponds (*Polypylis*, *Hippeutis*, *Planorbis*)	Cercariae encyst as metacercariae on herbage	Man, Pig
Heterophyes heterophyes	Lakes, ponds and streams (*Pirenella*, *Cerithidea*)	Cercariae encyst as metacercariae in freshwater fish	Man, Carnivores
Metagonimus yokogawai	Lakes, ponds and streams (*Semisulcospira*)	Cercariae encyst as metacercariae in freshwater fish	Man, Carnivores
Dicrocoelium dendriticum	Dry pastures (*Helicella*, *Zebrina*)	Cercariae encyst as metacercariae in ants	Sheep (Man?)
Gastrodiscoides hominis	Ponds (*Helicorbis*)	Cercariae encyst as metacercariae on herbage	Pigs, Man
Echinostomes	Ponds and lakes (*Planorbids*)	Cercariae encyst as metacercariae in freshwater fish	Mammals, Birds (Man)

Fig. 2.2 Intermediate hosts of trematodes.

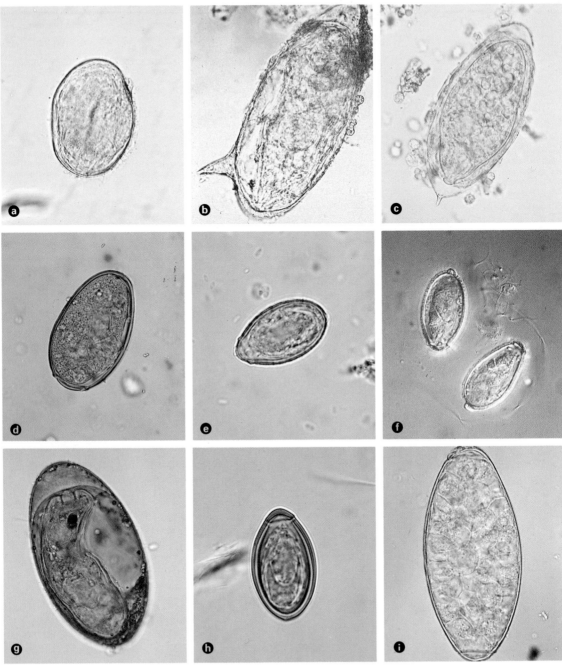

Fig. 2.3 Eggs of trematodes: (a) *Schistosoma japonicum* × 400. All schistosome eggs contain a miracidium. (b) *S. mansoni* × 400. (c) *S. haematobium* × 400. The egg of *S. intercalatum* is similar. (d) *Paragonimus westermani* × 400. Unembryonated. (e) *Clonorchis sinensis* × 1000. Contains miracidium. (f) *Opisthorchis viverrini* × 1000. Contains miracidium. (g) *Fasciolopsis buski* × 400. This egg has been kept in water for 5 weeks and therefore contains a miracidium; it is usually unembryonated. Contents usually similar to *Paragonimus westermani*. The egg of *Fasciola hepatica* is identical. (h) *Heterophyes heterophyes* × 1000. The egg of *Metagonimus yokogawai* is very similar. Contains a miracidium. (j) *Gastrodiscoides hominis* × 400. Unembryonated.

A ciliated miracidium larva hatches from the egg (Figs 2.3 & 2.4), enters a snail and develops into a sac-like sporocyst. Germ-cells inside this primary sporocyst form secondary larval stages which burst out and invade new tissues of the snail, usually the digestive gland. Here they develop into either rediae, with a primitive gut, or secondary sporocysts. Germ cells inside these develop into tailed cercariae which escape from the snail into the water.

Species	Egg size (μm)
Schistosoma japonicum	85 × 60
S. mansoni	140 × 60
S. haematobium	130 × 62
Paragonimus westermani	90 × 55
Clonorchis sinensis	25 × 15
Opisthorchis viverrini	25 × 15
Fasciolopsis buski and *F. hepatica*	140 × 80
Heterophyes heterophyes	30 × 15
Gastrodiscoides hominis	160 × 65

Fig. 2.4 Relative sizes of trematode eggs.

SCHISTOSOMA

Causative organism	Disease
Schistosoma japonicum	Intestinal schistosomiasis
Schistosoma mansoni	Intestinal schistosomiasis
Schistosoma haematobium	Urinary schistosomiasis
Schistosoma intercalatum	Intestinal schistosomiasis

The blood flukes or schistosomes give rise to a group of the most important helminth diseases of man; there are over 200 million cases of schistosomiasis (bilharziasis) in the world, with a mortality rate of 4.4 per million persons infected and an annual economic loss reckoned at $0.8 billion. The schistosomes differ from other trematodes as the sexes are separate; the male has a groove or gynaecophoric canal in which the longer but more slender female is held during copulation and oviposition (Fig. 2.5).

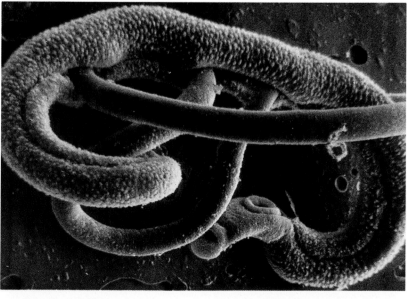

Fig. 2.5 Scanning electron micrograph of adult male (larger) and female *Schistosoma mansoni*.

Transmission and epidemiology

Schistosomiasis is primarily a rural disease, particularly affecting agricultural communities and, in Africa, fishermen (Fig. 2.6). The distribution and ecological factors associated with transmission of the human schistosomes vary with the habitat of the snail intermediate hosts. The amphibian snail hosts of *S. japonicum* live principally in rice paddies and on the muddy banks of rivers in the Far East. The aquatic snail hosts of *S. mansoni* live in slowly flowing water such as irrigation channels, streams and lakes in Africa, South America and the West Indies. Those transmitting *S. haematobium* and *S. intercalatum* live almost entirely in still water such as ponds, pools and lakes in Africa. The construction of dams in Africa is increasing the incidence of schistosomiasis in many countries.

Man is the only definitive host for *S. haematobium* and *S. intercalatum* but *S. japonicum* often occurs in cattle, dogs and rats, and *S. mansoni* can develop in baboons in Africa and rodents in South America.

The life cycle of *Schistosoma* is illustrated in Fig. 2.7. Eggs are passed in the faeces (or the urine in the case of *S. haematobium*) and each egg contains a fully formed miracidium larva which hatches out when the egg reaches water (Fig. 2.8). For further development, the ciliated larva must penetrate a suitable species of gastropod snail (*see* Fig. 2.9). Inside the snail, a process of asexual multiplication occurs giving primary and secondary sporocysts until many thousands of the next free-living stage, the fork-tailed cercariae, emerge after 4–7 weeks. The cercariae swim around in the water and infect man by penetrating the skin. The immature schistosomes are carried in the lymph to the lungs and reach the portal vessels. Here they grow to maturity and mate; the adult worms pair, then migrate against the blood flow to the posterior mesenteric veins (or the veins of the vesical plexus in the case of *S. haematobium*).

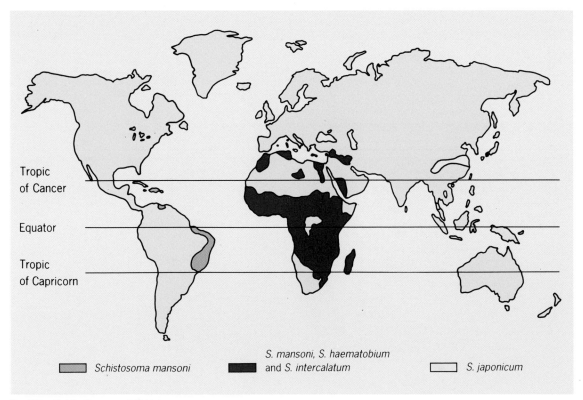

Fig. 2.6 Distribution map of *Schistosoma*.

Egg production begins 4–8 weeks after infection and the adult worms normally live for 2–5 years, although they can sometimes survive much longer. Eggs escape by penetrating venule walls, then the wall of the colon (or bladder in the case of *S. haematobium*) to the lumen and emerging with the faeces (or urine for *S. haematobium*).

Clinical effects

Penetration of cercariae after primary exposure usually causes a transient dermatitis; 'swimmer's itch'. Infection with *S. japonicum* can cause acute allergic manifestations when eggs are first produced, including pyrexia, lymphadenopathy, splenomegaly and diarrhoea ('Katayama syndrome') with high eosinophilia and liver tenderness.

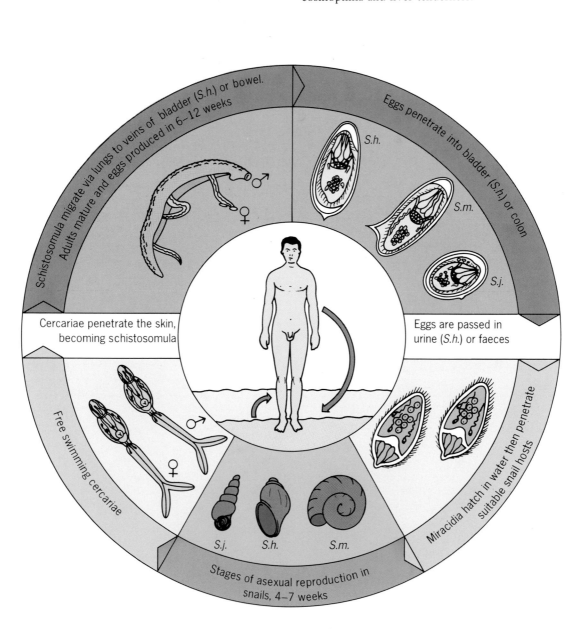

Fig. 2.7 Life cycle of *Schistosoma*.

In light infections there are few if any clinical effects during the chronic phase. In heavy infections, however, many eggs do not reach the lumen of the large intestine (or bladder in the case of *S. haematobium*) and become trapped in the tissues. Here they are surrounded by inflammatory cells, forming characteristic pseudotubercles (see Fig. 5.6); these coalesce to form larger granulomatous reactions (polyps) and the eggs eventually calcify (Fig. 2.10). Numerous polyps in the colon and rectum can cause a life-threatening dysentery with loss of fluids and blood, particularly common in Egypt.

Eggs carried to the liver in the portal veins can eventually lead to Symmer's 'clay pipe stem' peri-portal fibroids in schistosomiasis japonicum and mansoni (Fig. 2.11). The resulting portal hypertension leads to liver and spleen enlargement and possibly ascites (Fig. 2.12), and a gross enlargement of the oesophageal and gastric veins (varices) which sometimes burst.

Eggs of *S. japonicum* are sometimes also carried to the brain or spinal cord. In the case of schistosomiasis haematobium, blood in the urine (haematuria) is very common and the progressive disruption of the bladder wall can occasionally lead to carcinoma. Fibrosis of the bladder wall with reduced capacity and lesions of the ureters can cause nephrosis and eventually renal failure. Eggs reaching the lungs

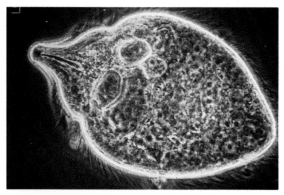

Fig. 2.8 Miracidium of *Schistosoma*.

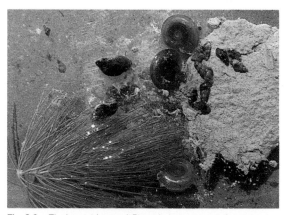

Fig. 2.9 The largest (orange) *Biomphalaria* transmit *S. mansoni*; the intermediate size *Bulinus* transmit *S. haematobium* and *S. intercalatum*; and the smallest, amphibious *Oncomelania* transmit *S. japonicum* (these do not occur together in nature).

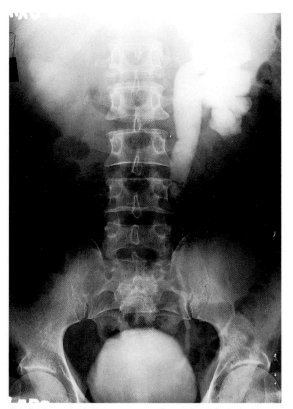

Fig. 2.10 Intravenous pyelogram of a woman infected with *S. hamatobium* showing hydronephrosis and calcification of the bladder. Courtesy of Dr D M Forsyth.

because of the collateral circulation by-passing the liver can cause pulmonary arteritis and even fatal heart failure. Clubbing of the fingers is one clinical sign of cor pulmonale.

Diagnosis

The most important method of diagnosis is finding eggs in the faeces or, for *S. haematobium*, in urine (often accompanied by haematuria). Concentration techniques such as the formol–ether method or filtration methods can be used, if necessary.

Rectal biopsy is often effective (even in 50 per cent of *S. haematobium* cases), the unstained squash being examined microscopically for eggs.

Immunodiagnostic tests are more useful in epidemiological surveys than for individual diagnosis: complement fixation and a micro-ELISA are most often employed.

Treatment

Praziquantel is effective against all species of schistosome in a single oral dose, with low toxicity and good tolerance, even in severe clinical cases.

Niridazole, given orally for a few days, is most effective against *S. haematobium* but has frequent, although not usually severe, side effects. Metrifonate is effective orally against *S. haematobium* with low toxicity.

Oxamniquine, in a single oral dose, is effective against *S. mansoni* only, with usually minor side effects.

Prevention and control

Visitors to endemic areas should avoid contact with water in possible transmission sites. For indigenous populations, there are five methods of control: prevention of water contact, mass chemotherapy, destruction of snails, alteration of habitats and sanitary disposal of faeces and urine (environmental sanitation). In many man-made habitats, snail control has proved most promising in the short term.

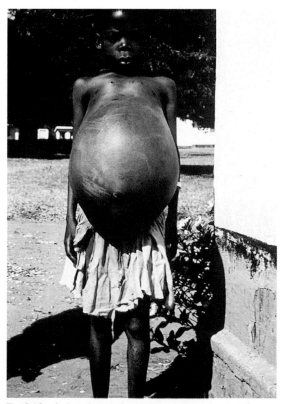

Fig. 2.12 A clinical case of schistosomiasis mansoni with marked hepatosplenomegaly and ascites. Courtesy of Prof. G Webbe.

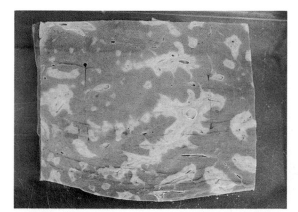

Fig. 2.11 Appearance of cut surface of infected liver showing the lighter Symmer's pipestem fibrosis surrounding the portal veins. The liver parenchymal cells are unaffected.

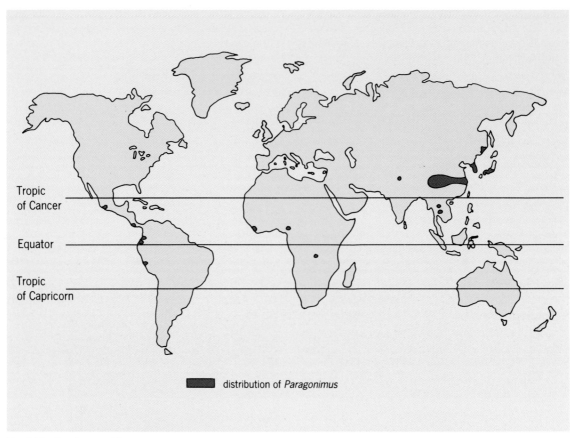

Fig. 2.13 Distribution of *Paragonimus*.

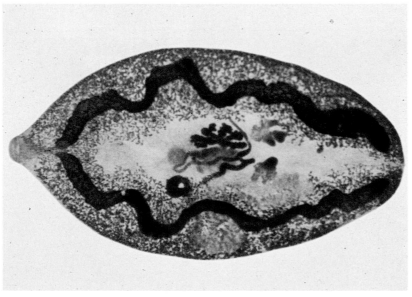

Fig. 2.14 Adult of *Paragonimus westermani* (stained specimen). It is about 12mm long, 5mm wide and 4mm thick. Courtesy of Dr S Vajrasthira.

PARAGONIMUS

Causative organism	Disease
Paragonimus westermani lung fluke	Paragonimiasis

Transmission and epidemiology

Species of *Paragonimus* are found in crustacean-eating carnivores in Asia, Africa and the Americas. Human cases are unusual except in the Far East where, for instance, there are over one million cases in Korea (Fig. 2.13).

The adults (Fig. 2.14) are thick, fleshy trematodes, measuring about 12mm in length and living as pairs in cysts in the lungs. The non-embryonated, brownish eggs produced (measuring 85–110 × 50–60μm) may escape in the sputum or the faeces after being swallowed (Fig. 2.15). If they reach water, a miracidium larva develops inside the egg, which hatches

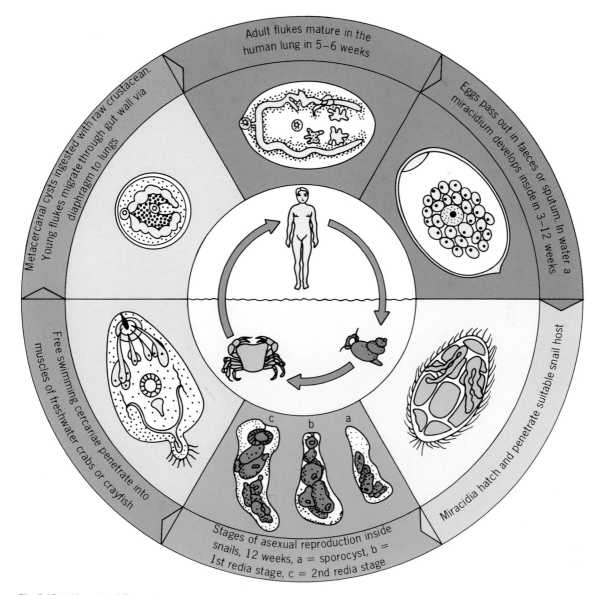

Adult flukes mature in the human lung in 5–6 weeks

Eggs pass out in faeces or sputum. In water a miracidium develops inside in 3–12 weeks

Miracidia hatch and penetrate suitable snail host

Stages of asexual reproduction inside snails, 12 weeks, a = sporocyst, b = 1st redia stage, c = 2nd redia stage

Free swimming cercariae penetrate into muscles of freshwater crabs or crayfish

Metacercarial cysts ingested with raw crustacean. Young flukes migrate through gut wall via diaphragm to lungs

Fig. 2.15 Life cycle of *Paragonimus*.

in about 3 weeks, and penetrates suitable, operculate, freshwater snails (*see* Fig. 2.2, p.59).

Asexual multiplication in the snail (producing sporocysts, then two generations of rediae) produces very short-tailed cercariae in three months; these penetrate into freshwater crabs or crayfish and encyst. If the crustacea are eaten raw as food, the young flukes burrow through the intestinal wall and diaphragm to the lungs (Fig. 2.16). Hermaphroditic adults lay eggs by six weeks and can live for many years.

In the Philippines, a dish, *kinagang*, is prepared from crab juice and in parts of China live crabs are eaten after steeping in rice wine. In Korea, children can become infected from swallowing crayfish juice as a cure for measles.

Clinical effects

The adult worms in the lungs provoke inflammatory and granulomatous reactions and the first effects are usually a dry cough, chest pain, difficulty in breathing and blood in the sputum (haemoptysis).

By three months after infection, there is 25 per cent eosinophilia and pairs of worms are found in cysts surrounded by an inflammatory reaction but with an opening into a bronchus. Cysts contain a brown, purulent fluid and in heavy infections can cause broncho-pneumonia with fever.

Adult worms may also migrate to the brain where they, and discharged eggs, become foci for abscesses developed from granulomas, resulting in symptoms similar to epilepsy, a cerebral tumour or embolism and sometimes causing paralysis. Many such cases are in children (Fig. 2.17).

Diagnosis

Eggs can be found in the rust-coloured sputum (often when looking for tubercle bacilli) or faeces but are often very scarce in chronic infections and so concentration techniques, for example, sedimentation with 2 per cent sodium hydroxide, are useful.

The complement fixation test works well but cross-reacts with schistosomiasis and clonorchiasis. Immunoelectrophoresis is more specific. X-rays show nodular or ring ('soap bubble') shadows, usually mistaken for tuberculosus.

Treatment

Praziquantel taken orally over three days is very effective and has few side effects. Bithionol can also be given orally over twenty days, rarely with serious side effects, but has no effect against migratory stages. For cerebral cases, surgery may be necessary and about 30 per cent of such cases are improved.

Prevention and control

Light cooking will kill the cysts in crustacea and care should be taken with cysts on hands, knives and

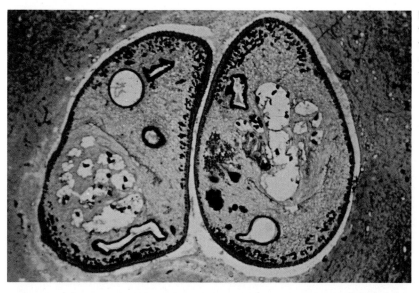

Fig. 2.16 A section of a lung cyst with two adult *Paragonimus*. Note fibrous cyst wall and two branches of the gut and central uterus inside the trematode. Courtesy of H Zaiman.

chopping boards. In Japan, where there are few animal reservoirs, sanitary improvements have lowered incidence in recent years.

About 27 species of *Paragonimus* occur in wild carnivores and occasional human cases have been reported from many countries. With some, adults do not develop and young stages wander around in the body causing a larva migrans.

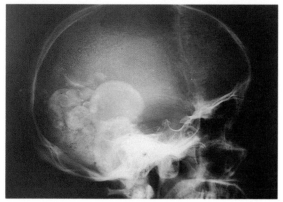

Fig. 2.17   Head X-radiograph of a girl with calcified cysts of *Paragonimus* in the occipital lobes. Courtesy of Y Matsukado.

CLONORCHIS **AND** *OPISTHORCHIS*

Causative organism	Disease
Clonorchis sinensis (Chinese liver fluke)	Clonorchiasis
Opisthorchis viverrini	Opisthorchiasis
Opisthorchis felineus	Opisthorchiasis

Transmission and epidemiology

Infection with *Clonorchis sinensis* and *Opisthorchis viverrini* is confined to the Far East; *Opisthorchis felineus* is normally found in the bile ducts of cats but human cases occur, principally in Poland, the Ukraine and Siberia (Fig. 2.18). The hermaphroditic adults measure 6–20mm in length and are extremely

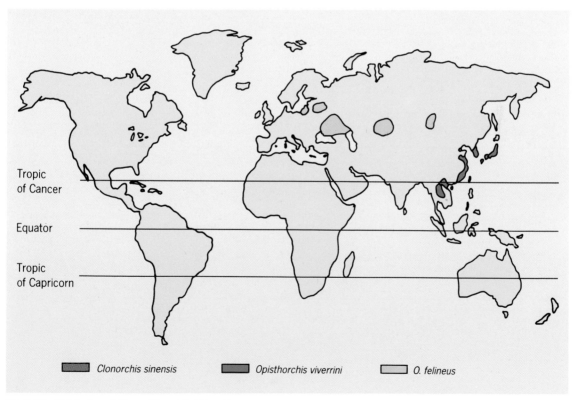

Clonorchis sinensis   Opisthorchis viverrini   O. felineus

Fig. 2.18   Distribution of *Clonorchis* and *Opisthorchis*.

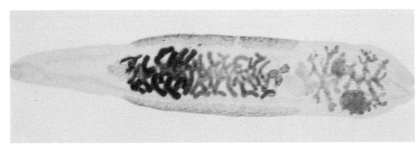

Fig. 2.19 An adult *Clonorchis sinensis* (stained specimen) measuring about 15mm long and 4mm wide.

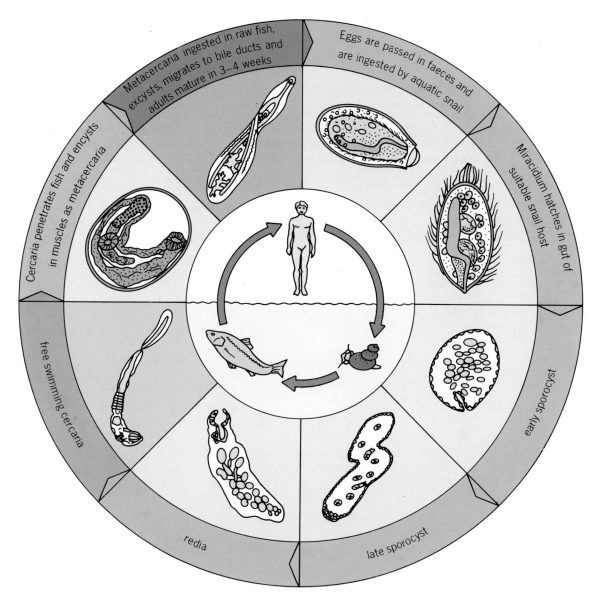

Fig. 2.20 Life cycle of *Clonorchis sinensis*.

flat; they inhabit the bile ducts, usually just under the liver capsule, but in heavy infections are found in the gall bladder and pancreatic ducts also. The adults of all are very similar but *Clonorchis* has branched and *Opisthorchis* lobed testes (Fig. 2.19).

The life cycle of *Clonorchis sinensis* is illustrated in Fig. 2.20. The small operculate eggs (23–35 × 10–20μm) are produced in large numbers and pass out in the faeces. If they reach fresh water and are ingested by a suitable operculate snail (see Fig. 2.2, p.59) the contained miracidium hatches and undergoes asexual multiplication (producing sporocysts and rediae), many cercariae emerging from the snail in a few weeks. Cercariae penetrate and encyst beneath the scales of freshwater fish. When fish are eaten raw or undercooked, the young flukes excyst and migrate up the bile ducts, maturing in 3–4 weeks, and adults can live many years.

Dogs are important reservoir hosts of *Clonorchis*, as are civet cats and domestic cats of *Opisthorchis*.

Clinical effects

Infection with *C. sinensis* is widespread in many endemic areas with sometimes over 70 per cent of the population being infected. The infection is usually light, with only a few worms present; however, more worms may be acquired progressively over the years so that the onset of clinical disease may be insidious and occurs principally in older age groups. Light infections are completely symptomless but the presence of hundreds or thousands of worms results in diarrhoea, painful liver enlargement and eosinophilia, followed by cholecystitis and possibly recurrent biliary colic with jaundice.

Adult trematodes provoke an intense inflammatory reaction of the bile duct wall (Fig. 2.21), followed in heavy infections by hyperplasia of the epithelium and perhaps the formation of new biliary ductules with destruction of the liver parenchyma. Over the years, recurrent cholangitis leads to widespread fibrosis of the bile ducts and may result in portal hypertension with splenomegaly. Carcinoma of the bile ducts (adenocarcinoma) may develop eventually (Fig. 2.22).

Diagnosis

Eggs are usually plentiful in the faeces but must be differentiated from other small trematode eggs. If scarce, concentration techniques or swallowing a brushed nylon string can be used.

In cases of recurrent pyogenic cholangitis, worms are killed by bacteria (usually *Escherichia coli*) present in the ducts and immunodiagnosis (for example, complement fixation) or clinical diagnosis is necessary.

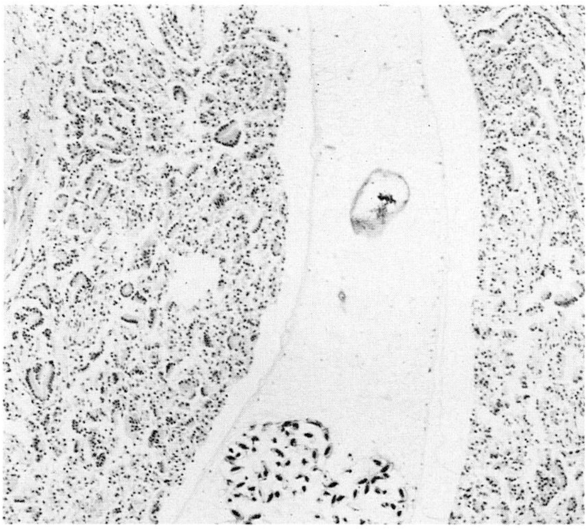

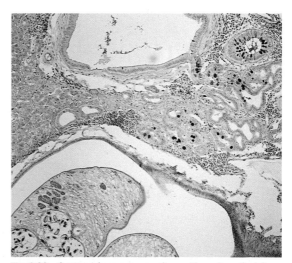

Fig. 2.21 Microscopic section of bile duct with adult *Clonorchis* in centre (uterus containing numerous eggs and cross-section of one gut caecum can be seen). Note the extensive proliferation and oedema of the bile duct epithelium.

Fig. 2.22 Section of precancerous liver with portion of adult *Opisthorchis viverrini* at bottom. Stained for mucin (blue) found in the goblet cells which are developing in abnormal areas (metaplasia), an early feature of adenocarcinoma. Courtesy of Dr D Flavell.

Treatment

Praziquantel taken orally for one day has given high cure rates with acceptable side effects. Albendazole given orally for three consecutive days cures about 85 per cent of cases with few side effects.

Control and prevention

Thorough cooking of fish will kill metacercarial cysts (Fig. 2.23), but raw fish is an important dietary item in many countries and cysts also get on knives and chopping boards.

Treatment of faeces before using as a fertilizer is now being practised in China and a control programme based on chemotherapy and community based health education is being operated in northeast Thailand where there are about 3.5 million cases of *O. viverrini* infection.

FASCIOLA

Causative organism	Disease
Fasciola hepatica	Fascioliasis

Transmission and epidemiology

Fasciola is a common parasite of sheep and cattle kept on damp pastures in many parts of the world but is only occasionally found in man. Most cases have been from South America, France, Western Britain and North Africa. In Europe, human outbreaks are associated with particularly wet summers.

The hermaphroditic adults measure 20–30mm, are much flattened and almost all organs are very highly branched (Fig. 2.24); they live in the bile ducts and each produces about 300 eggs daily. The large, undifferentiated eggs (140 × 80μm) pass out in the faeces of sheep and cattle. A miracidium develops in each and after hatching out can reach a suitable snail by swimming in a film of moisture on wet pasture. Inside the snail, there is asexual multiplication (producing sporocysts and two redial stages) and the cercariae which emerge in 4–5 weeks encyst as metacercariae on vegetation (usually grass, but water cress or radishes in the case of human infection). When cysts are ingested the young flukes penetrate the duodenum wall and reach the bile ducts by eating their way through the liver tissue (Fig. 2.25).

Very few human cases of infection with *Fasciola gigantica* of cattle and other herbivores in Africa, Asia and the Pacific have been reported. The snail hosts live in ponds, so contaminated vegetation is not likely to be eaten by man, although the parasite is of great economic importance in livestock.

Clinical effects

Symptoms of dyspepsia, nausea, fever and

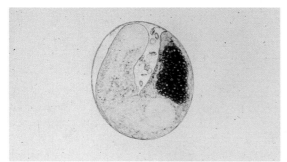

Fig. 2.23 Metacercaria of *Clonorchis* removed from muscles of fish.

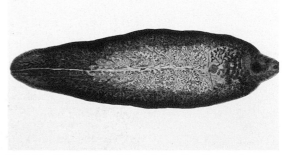

Fig. 2.24 Stained adult of *Fasciola hepatica*. Almost all systems are highly branched, including the gut caeca.

abdominal pain, accompanied by a high eosinophilia, characterise the acute phase while the young flukes are migrating through the liver tissues.

The chronic phase ensues when they reach the bile ducts and there is often painful liver enlargement and perhaps an obstructive jaundice resembling biliary disease. The bile ducts can be severely damaged and there may be some anaemia. Later there is a marked biliary fibrosis (Fig. 2.25 lower).

Diagnosis

Eggs in the faeces are often scarce or non-existent and duodenal aspiration or swallowing a brushed nylon string in a gelatine capsule (enterotest) may help to find them.

The passive haemagglutination and complement fixation tests are a sensitive means of diagnosis.

Treatment

Bithionol is given orally for 10–15 days, or in a single dose, and only rarely has serious side effects.

Control and prevention

Sheep or cattle faeces should not be allowed near watercress beds in streams. Infection in domestic stock is an important economic problem worldwide and can be controlled by draining fields to prevent snails, by mollusciciding and by chemotherapy for livestock.

FASCIOLOPSIS

Causative organism	Disease
Fasciolopis buski Busk's fluke	Fasciolopsiasis

Transmission and epidemiology

The largest endemic foci of infection are in Central and South China but fasciolopsiasis also occurs in other parts of Asia. The large adult trematodes (Fig. 2.26), measuring 20–75mm in length, are found in the small intestine. The eggs (measuring 140 ×

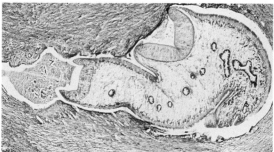

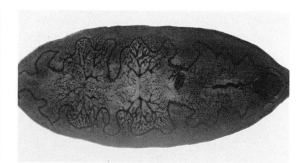

Fig. 2.25 Section of bile duct and liver with two cross-sections of *Fasciola hepatica*. The epithelium has been destroyed and the duct wall thickened. Many branches of the gut of the trematode can be seen (upper). Section of *Fasciola* through oral and ventral suckers to show fibrosis (stained blue) of bile duct wall (lower).

Fig. 2.26 Stained adult of *Fasciolopsis buski*, showing highly branched testes and ovary but two simple gut caeca. Courtesy of Dr S Vajrasthira.

80μm and similar to those of *Fasciola*) pass out in the faeces and the emergent miracidia enter suitable snail hosts (see Fig. 2.2).

The cercariae, which develop in the snails after the usual asexual multiplication (producing sporocysts and two redial stages), encyst on the fruits and roots of water plants, such as the water caltrop, water chestnut and lotus. The outer covering of these are often removed with the teeth, particularly by children.

The cysts are very susceptible to drying, so heavy infections are usually found in communities living close to infected ponds. Pigs (hogs) act as important reservoir hosts.

Clinical effects

In most cases infection is light and there are no symptoms but when many worms are present there is nausea, diarrhoea and intense griping pains in the morning, relieved by food. A characteristic facial oedema may also occur with other signs of generalized allergy.

The adult worms can cause traumatic inflammatory damage to the mucosa at the site of attachment of the large ventral sucker, with an excessive production of mucus.

Diagnosis

Diagnosis is made by recovery of eggs in the faeces, using concentration techniques if necessary, although over 20 000 are produced daily by each worm.

Treatment

Praziquantel in a single oral dose is very effective. Tetrachlorethylene, in a single oral dose is still used because of cheapness, although causing numerous side effects. Clinical treatment of any associated toxaemia should also be undertaken if necessary.

Prevention and control

Water vegetables should be carefully peeled and washed. Boiling for a few seconds will kill the metacercariae cysts.

Human faeces should be treated before being used as fertilizer in ponds and pig faeces should be kept away from ponds. Pigs should not be fed fresh water plants without their being dried first.

HETEROPHYES AND *METAGONIMUS*

Causative organism	Disease
Heterophyes heterophyes (dwarf fluke)	Heterophyiasis
Metagonimus yokogawai (Yokogawa's fluke)	Metagonimiasis

Transmission and epidemiology

These are very similar, minute trematodes, measuring 1–2mm, which attach themselves to the wall of the small intestine, between the villi (Fig. 2.27). *Heterophyes* is found in the Middle East (particularly Egypt), southern Europe and Asia, while *Metagonimus* is found only in Asia. Eggs (measuring 30 × 15μm) are passed via faeces into water and, if ingested by suitable snails, multiply inside them (through the stages of miracidia, sporocysts, rediae), the emergent cercariae encysting in freshwater fish.

Both parasites have a wide range of reservoir hosts and other members of the same family are occasionally found in man.

Clinical effects

In heavy infections, there is nausea, mucus diarrhoea and colicky pains. There may be mild inflammation and necrosis of the mucosa.

Diagnosis

Eggs in the faeces must be differentiated from those of *Clonorchis* and *Opisthorchis*.

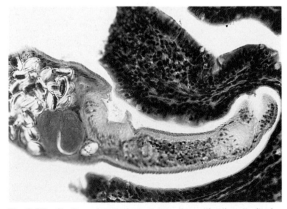

Fig. 2.27 Section of wall of small intestine with a longitudinal section of adult *Heterophyes heterophyes* showing oral and ventral suckers and portion of uterus containing eggs.

Treatment

Albendazole, given orally over two days, is moderately effective with few side effects. Niclosamide, given orally over 2–3 days, cures about 80 per cent of cases. Praziquantel, in a single oral dose, is probably effective but needs further evaluation.

Control and prevention

Adequate cooking of fish will kill the cysts.

GASTRODISCOIDES

Causative organism	Disease
Gastrodiscoides hominis	Gastrodisciasis

Transmission and epidemiology

Human infection is found in India (Assam), Bangladesh, Vietnam, China, the Philippines and Russia.

Adult *Gastrodiscoides* measure 5–14mm in length and have a discoidal, posterior part and a conical anterior end. They attach to the wall of the colon or caecum. Large, unembryonated eggs (160 × 65μm) are passed in the faeces. Miracidia develop inside and, after emerging, search for a suitable snail host. Cercariae encyst on vegetation.

Clinical effects

In heavy infections, there may be a mucus diarrhoea with superficial inflammation of the mucosa.

Diagnosis

Diagnosis is made by identifying eggs in faeces.

Treatment

Praziquantel would probably be effective but has not been evaluated.

Control and prevention

Water caltrop is often involved, and all water vegetables should be carefully peeled and washed. Boiling for a few seconds will kill metacercarial cysts.

Pigs act as important reservoir hosts, and therefore pig faeces should be kept away from ponds. Water plants should be dried before being fed to pigs.

THE CESTODES

All adult cestodes inhabit the intestinal tract. They differ from trematodes in having a flat tape-like body, lacking a gut and are made up of hermaphroditic segments known as proglottids, the whole chain being called a strobila (Fig. 2.28).

All cestodes of man, except *Diphyllobothrium*, belong to the order Cyclophyllidea and have an anterior scolex or hold-fast organ, usually with hooks, and undifferentiated neck region. This is followed by mature proglottids in which male

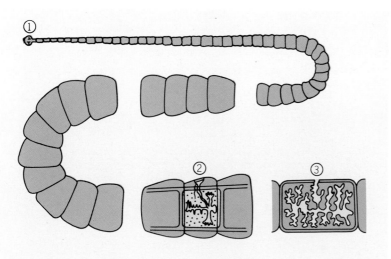

Fig. 2.28 Typical cestode features as exemplified by *Taenia* spp; 1, scolex; 2, mature proglottids; 3, gravid proglottids.

organs are functional, then mature proglottids in which female organs are functional. Finally, there are gravid proglottids containing a uterus filled with eggs, which detach and pass out of the body (Fig. 2.28).

Diphyllobothrium belongs to the order Pseudophyllidea which differs from Cyclophyllidea in that the scolex has two sucking grooves and also has differences in the life cycle. Adult tapeworm infections are usually more unpleasant than serious but larval infections can be life-threatening public health problems.

DIPHYLLOBOTHRIUM LATUM

Causative organism	Disease
Diphyllobothrium latum (broad fish tapeworm)	Diphyllobothriasis

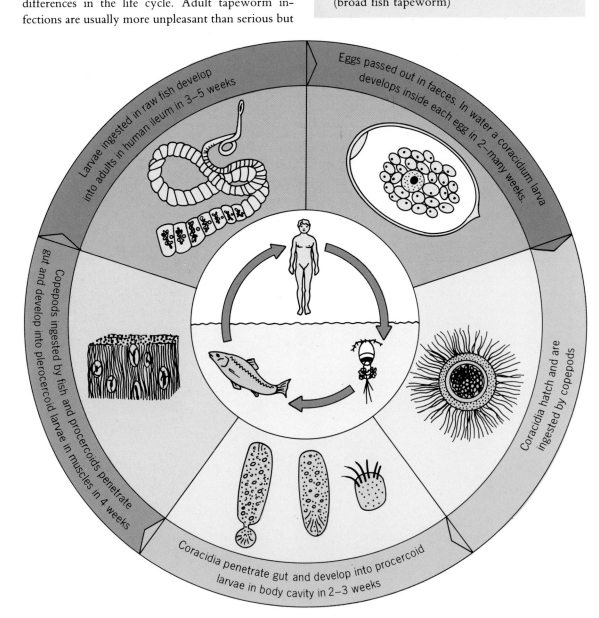

Fig. 2.29 Life cycle of *Diphyllobothrium latum*.

Transmission and epidemiology

Infection by *Diphyllobothrium latum* occurs in temperate and subarctic countries with many lakes, where fish are eaten raw, such as Finland, USSR, Central Europe, Japan, the Great Lakes regions of Canada and USA, and Chile.

The life cycle of *D. latum* is shown in Fig. 2.29. It is the longest tapeworm infecting man, measuring 3–10m in length and with up to 4000 proglottids. The scolex of the adult tapeworm is attached to the wall of the small intestine, by the two sucking grooves (Fig. 2.30), with the rest of the tape extending throughout its length. Each proglottid has both male and female reproductive organs with a uterine pore through which eggs are discharged; a single worm may produce one million eggs daily. The operculate, unsegmented eggs measure about 65 × 45μm and are passed out in the faeces (Fig. 2.31).

After reaching fresh water, a ciliated coracidium larva develops in the egg, emerges in a few weeks and needs to be ingested by a suitable planktonic microcrustacean (*Diaptomus* or *Cyclops*). Inside the body cavity, it changes to a procercoid larva (Fig. 2.32), and, if the microcrustacean is ingested by a freshwater fish, the larva penetrates the intestinal wall and develops to a plerocercoid larva in the muscles. Larvae can be transferred from small species to larger carnivorous fish (for example, trout and pike).

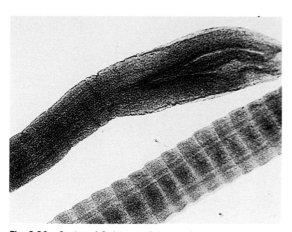

Fig. 2.30 Scolex of *D. latum* with two sucking grooves.

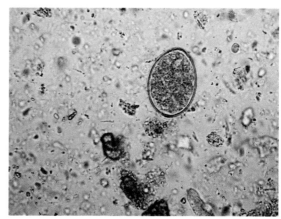

Fig. 2.31 Egg of *D. latum*.

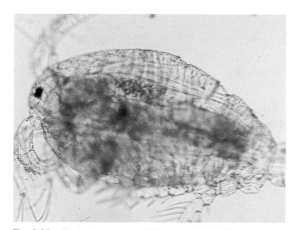

Fig. 2.32 First-stage procercoid larvae inside *Cyclops*, a freshwater crustacean.

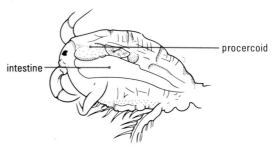

intestine

procercoid

Clinical effects

There are usually none, apart from eosinophilia in the early stages, but there may be abdominal pain, dizziness, fatigue, diarrhoea, vomiting and numbness of the extremities. In Finland, a characteristic tapeworm anaemia used to be common. This was of the pernicious megaloblastic (macrocytic) type, caused by competitive uptake of dietary vitamin B_{12} by the worm. This is now rare, probably because of a better winter diet, coupled with better health care (particularly prenatal care) and treatment.

Fig. 2.33 Life cycles of *Taenia solium* and *T. saginata*.

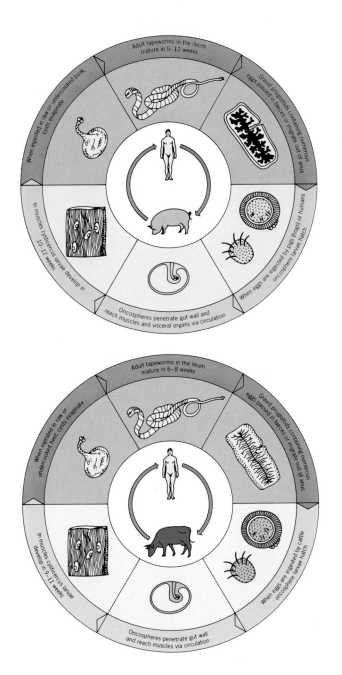

Diagnosis

There are usually numerous eggs in the faeces and sometimes chains of proglottids are passed; these can be recognized by the rosette-shaped uterus filled with brown eggs.

Treatment

Praziquantel or niclosamide, given orally as a single dose in the morning, are both very effective. Bithionol in a single oral dose can also be used. Vitamin B_{12} should be given, after curative treatment, to all patients.

Prevention and control

The plerocercoid larvae in fish are killed by cooking, freezing or thorough pickling.

The proper treatment of sewage before adding to lakes, combined with effective chemotherapy, has

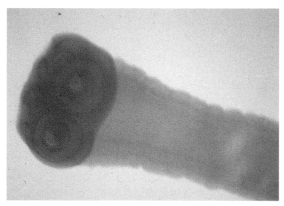

Fig. 2.34   Scolex of *T. saginata* showing 4 suckers but no hooks.

greatly reduced the incidence in Finland in the last few years.

TAENIA

Causative organism	Disease
Taenia saginata (beef tapeworm)	Taeniasis

Transmission and epidemiology

The life cycle is outlined in Fig. 2.33. Infection by *Taenia saginata* is cosmopolitan and occurs where beef is eaten raw or lightly cooked. The scolex of the adult tapeworm (Fig. 2.34) is attached to the wall of the ileum by four suckers (both the cysticerci and adults lack the typical taeniid hooks), with the rest of the 5–20m long tape extended throughout the small intestine.

Both male and female organs develop in each proglottid but unlike *Diphyllobothrium* there is no uterine pore, so the ultimate gravid proglottids containing a branched uterus filled with eggs (Fig. 2.35) (measuring 43–47μm in diameter) drop off and are usually passed intact out of the anus. The eggs (Fig. 2.36) which reach the ground are very resistant to drying and sewage treatment, and can live for weeks on pastures. If they are ingested by cattle, however, the contained larvae (oncospheres) hatch in the duodenum and penetrate the wall to reach the muscles via the circulation. They develop into fluid-filled cysticerci larvae, measuring 8mm, in about 12

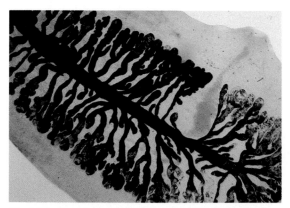

Fig. 2.35   Gravid proglottids of *T. saginata*. The uterus has been stained with Indian ink to show number of side branches.

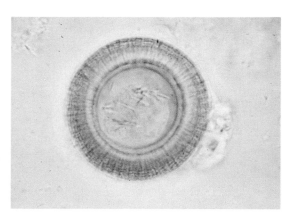

Fig. 2.36   Egg of *T. saginata* containing 6-hooked hexacanth larva. That of *T. solium* is identical.

weeks in the muscles (known to veterinarians as cysticercus bovis) (Fig. 2.37). Each will develop into an adult tapeworm when ingested by man.

Clinical effects
Infection is frequently asymptomatic, the first sign being the presence of gravid proglottids in the faeces, or crawling out through the anus: symptoms often begin once these are perceived.

Symptoms may include abdominal pain, nausea and headache, or occasionally generalized allergic manifestations such as urticaria with anal pruritis. Attachment of the scolex rarely causes inflammation of the intestinal mucosa. A few cases of intestinal obstruction have been reported.

Diagnosis
A few highly active proglottids are passed out at intervals and, when pressed between glass slides, the presence and number of lateral branches (15–32) of the uterus can usually identify the species. Eggs may be found in the faeces in about 50 per cent of cases.

Treatment
Praziquantel, in a single oral dose, appears to have a 100 per cent cure rate. Albendazole and niclosamide, given in single oral doses, are also very effective.

Prevention and control
Thorough cooking (above 56°C) of beef will kill the cysts. Meat inspection for the white pin-head sized cysts ('measly beef') is the most important public health measure, although adequate treatment of sewage is very important.

Causative organism	Disease
Taenia solium (pork tapeworm)	Taeniasis

Transmission and epidemiology
The distribution of *Taenia solium* is confined to countries where pork or pork products are eaten raw or undercooked. Infection is most common in Eastern Europe, Mexico, Chile, South Africa, China and Indonesia.

The scolex of *T. solium* (Fig. 2.38) becomes embedded in the mucosa of the small intestine by means of the four suckers and two rows of typical taeniid hooks, with the rest of the 2–10m long tape extending through the ileum. Mature segments are similar to those of *T. saginata*. Gravid proglottids (Fig. 2.39) with 7–13 side branches to the uterus containing numerous eggs, are passed out in the faeces. The eggs are identical to those of *T. saginata* (43–47μm in diameter) and are also very resistant.

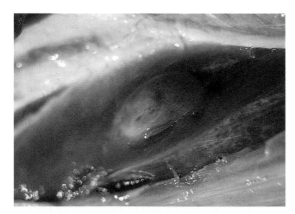

Fig. 2.37 Encysted larva of *T. saginata* (cysticercus bovis) in muscles of cow, measuring 7mm and with no hooks on the prototoscolex. Courtesy of Dr P Stevenson.

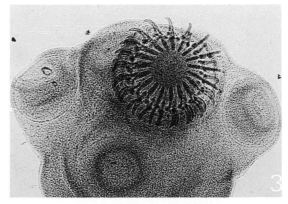

Fig. 2.38 Scolex of *T. solium* with 4 suckers and 2 rows of taeniid type hooks. Courtesy of Dr M Colbourne.

The pig (hog) acts as the intermediate host and ingests eggs (or gravid proglottids) in faeces or soil. The contained onchosphere larvae hatch out in the duodenum, penetrate the wall and are carried to the voluntary muscles in the circulation. They form cysts (known to veterinarians as cysticerci cellulosae) measuring 8mm in about 70 days. Each consists of a hollow bladder with a small protoscolex, invaginated into the lumen, which has four suckers and two rows of hooks (Fig. 2.40). When infected pork or pork dishes are eaten raw or undercooked, each cysticercus can develop into an adult tapeworm in about 10 weeks.

Clinical effects
The presence of one or more adult tapeworms usually causes no distinct symptoms, but there may be vague abdominal pains, with diarrhoea or constipation, and a slight eosinophilia. There is superficial, traumatic damage at the site of attachment of the scolex. Human infection with the cysticerci of *T. solium* is also possible (see p.83) and this is much more serious.

Diagnosis
The presence of gravid proglottids or eggs in the faeces is the usual method: the former are not so active as those of *T. saginata* and can usually be differentiated by having fewer (7–13) main branches to the uterus.

Treatment
Praziquantel or niclosamide as for *T. saginata*.

Prevention and control
Thorough cooking of pork (pickling is not usually effective) and sanitary disposal of human faeces are required. Inspection of killed pigs in the abbatoir for the white, pin-head sized cysts (measly pork) is important.

HYMENOLEPIS

Causative organism	Disease
Hymenolepis nana (dwarf tapeworm)	Hymenolepiasis

Transmission and epidemiology
Infection by *Hymenolepis nana* is cosmopolitan, often occurring in children in institutions, and is most common in eastern and southern Europe, South America, and areas of Asia.

The small adult tapeworms (15–40mm long and with about 200 proglottids) inhabit the small

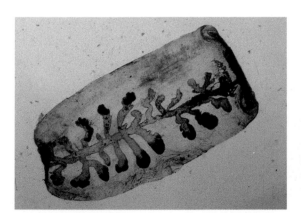

Fig. 2.39 Gravid proglottid of *T. solium*. The uterus has been stained with Indian ink to show the number of side branches.

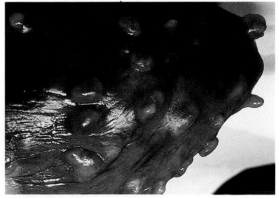

Fig. 2.40 Encysted larvae of *T. solium* (cysticerci cellulosae) in heart of pig. The protoscolices have hooks. Courtesy of Dr C D Mackenzie.

intestine with the scolex (Fig. 2.41) embedded in the mucosa by means of the four suckers and row of hooks. Gravid proglottids break up in the large intestine and eggs measuring $45 \times 30\mu m$ (Fig. 2.42) pass out in the faeces: they are immediately infective. If ingested by another person, the onchosphere is liberated in the small intestine and penetrates a villus (Fig. 2.43). It develops into a solid larva, known as a cysticercoid, which emerges into the lumen again after a few days to form the adult tapeworm.

H. nana is the only tapeworm known which does not require an intermediate host.

Clinical effects

In light infections, there are no specific symptoms but with over 2000 worms there may be enteritis, with symptoms of diarrhoea, vomiting, dizziness and abdominal pain. Autoinfection is common, so

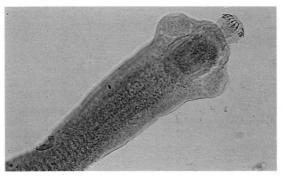

Fig. 2.41 Scolex of *Hymenolepis nana* with 4 suckers and a single row of hooks (these can be retracted into the scolex). It is considerably smaller than that of taeniid tapeworms.

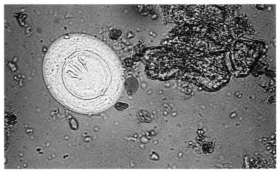

Fig. 2.42 Egg of *H. nana* containing 6-hooked hexacanth larva.

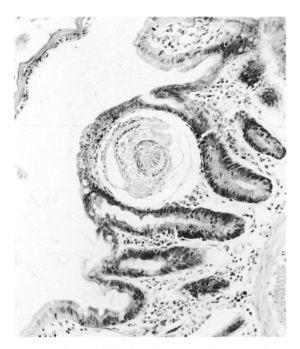

Fig. 2.43 Section of villi of small intestine with cysticercoid larva of *H. nana* under mucosa. This is the only tapeworm not requiring an intermediate host.

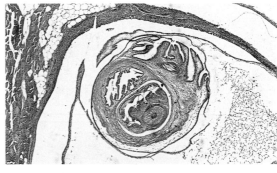

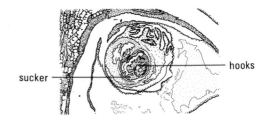

Fig. 2.44 Section of cysticercus of *T. solium* showing suckers and hooks.

that there can be a build-up of infection with perhaps many thousands of adult worms present.

Diagnosis

Diagnosis is made by identifying eggs in the faeces (gravid proglottids usually break up in the large intestine).

Treatment

Praziquantel in a single oral dose is very effective against adults, but not against young cysticercoids, so a second course of therapy is sometimes necessary. Niclosamide can also be given orally every day for a week.

Prevention and control

Infection is usually from hand to mouth, although it can be by food or water and is particularly common in institutions and children's homes. The eggs, however, are not resistant to dessication. *H. nana* is also found in the domestic mouse but the mouse strain does not appear to infect man.

OTHER TAPEWORMS

Hymenolepis diminuta is a common tapeworm of rats and mice and in some areas is a parasite of children. The adult measures about 400mm in length, with 1000 proglottids; the scolex has no hooks. Eggs (measuring 70μm in diameter) are passed in the faeces and need to be ingested by rat fleas or flour beetles, in which tailed cysticercoids develop: the ingested insects act as intermediate hosts. Infection in children causes no symptoms apart from diarrhoea.

Diagnosis is by finding eggs in the faeces and treatment is as for *H. nana*.

Dipylidium caninum is a cosmopolitan parasite of dogs and cats, and there have been about 200 asymptomatic cases reported from children. Dog fleas act as intermediate hosts.

LARVAL CESTODES

Causative organism	Disease
Taenia solium cysticerus	Cysticercosis

Transmission and epidemiology

Cysticercosis occurs in all areas where the adult tapeworm infection is common, particularly in South and Central America, China and Indonesia. Human infection takes place by the accidental ingestion of eggs of *T. solium* passed in human faeces, either on vegetables or in drinking water. It is not proven whether auto-infection from regurgitation of gravid proglottids into the stomach by anti-peristalsis ever occurs. When eggs are ingested, the contained oncosphere larvae hatch in the small intestine, penetrate the wall and are carried in the circulation all over the body, most commonly to the muscles or connective tissues, where they form cysticerci as in the pig.

Clinical effects

Clinical disease is usually caused by the presence of cysts in the brain or eyes (Fig. 2.46). Symptoms depend on the sites of the focal lesions but often include Jacksonian-type epilepsiform

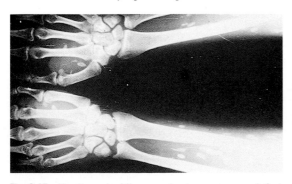

Fig. 2.45 X-radiograph of forearms showing numerous calcified cysts of *T. solium*.

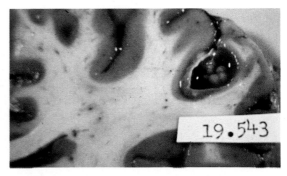

Fig. 2.46 Brain of man cut across to show a cyst of *T. solium*. This is the most serious manifestation of human cysticercosis. Courtesy of Prof. D B Holliman.

seizures. Headaches can be very severe and there may also be unconsciousness without convulsions.

Diagnosis

Subcutaneous nodules can often be seen and felt, and the diagnosis confirmed by biopsy. X-rays or computerized tomography scans can detect cysts which have calcified. The ELISA test can be used for serological diagnosis and, with new purified antigens, is fairly specific.

Treatment

Praziquantel, given orally every day for 1–2 weeks, is the standard treatment. Albendazole is also proving effective.

Prevention and control

Individual prevention is difficult, apart from thoroughly washing salad vegetables and strict personal hygiene. Control measures are the same as for the adult tapeworm, including sanitary disposal of faeces and inspection of pork.

Causative organism	Disease
Echinococcus granulosus	Echinococcosis (hydatidosis in animals)

Transmission and epidemiology

Echinococcus granulosus is found in most sheep and cattle raising areas of the world (Fig. 2.47). The highest prevalence of infection in man occurs among pastoral communities; highest prevalence rates (up to 0.1 per cent) are from Chile, Uruguay, North Kenya South Vietnam and China. There is marked geographical strain variation in *E. granulosus* and in

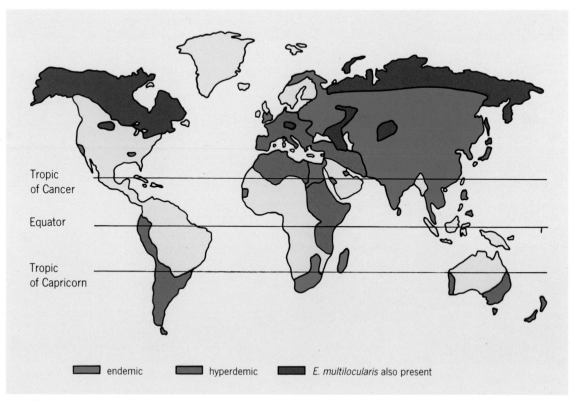

endemic   hyperdemic   *E. multilocularis* also present

Fig. 2.47 Distribution map of *Echinococcus granulosus*.

many areas cycles involving cattle or horses as intermediate hosts do not appear to be infective to man.

The minute adult tapeworm measures less than one centimetre in length. It has 3–5 proglottids and inhabits the small intestine of carnivores, such as the dog. There may be many thousands of worms

attached to the mucosa by the four suckers and two rows of hooks.

The life cycle of *E. granulosus* is illustrated in Fig. 2.48. The minute adult tapeworm measures less than one centimetre in length. It has 3–5 proglottids and inhabits the small intestine of carnivores, such as the

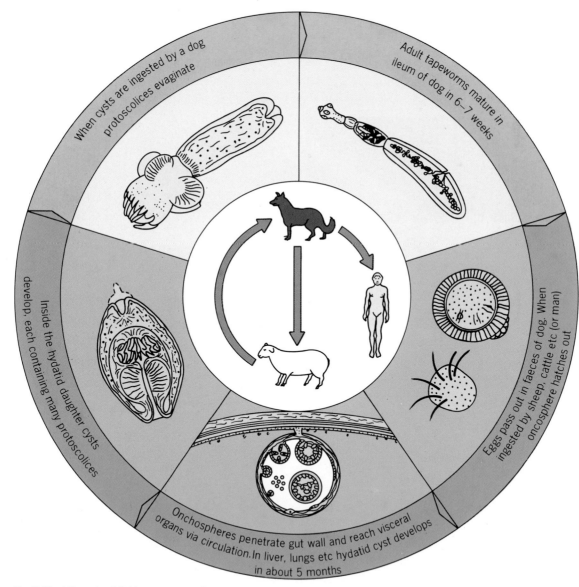

Fig. 2.48 Life cycle of *Echinococcus granulosus*.

Text around the figure (clockwise):

- Adult tapeworms mature in ileum of dog in 6–7 weeks
- Eggs pass out in faeces of dog. When ingested by sheep, cattle etc (or man) oncosphere hatches out
- Onchospheres penetrate gut wall and reach visceral organs via circulation. In liver, lungs etc hydatid cyst develops in about 5 months
- Inside the hydatid daughter cysts develop, each containing many protoscolices
- When cysts are ingested by a dog protoscolices evaginate

dog (Fig. 2.49). There may be many thousands of worms attached to the mucosa by the four suckers and two rows of hooks. A gravid proglottid detaches and eggs (measuring 35μm in diameter and appearing identical to most other taeniid eggs) are passed in the faeces. These are very resistant and can survive for months on pasture. When ingested by a suitable intermediate host, such as sheep, cattle, goat, camel or man, the released oncospheres penetrate the intestinal wall and are carried in the circulatory system to all parts of the body, but settle most frequently in the liver as they are filtered out in the portal capillaries. They can, however, also invade the lungs, brain and long bones. A slow-growing cyst develops which can eventually reach a size of 30cm in diameter after a few years. The 1mm thick cyst wall is laminated and usually surrounded by a fibrous host

tissue reaction. There is an inner germinative layer from which proliferate numerous bud-like protoscoleces with hooks and suckers and thin-walled daughter brood capsules containing protoscoleces which drop off into the fluid-filled cyst cavity. These mature cysts are ingested with offal by dogs in cycles involving domestic livestock or by wild carnivores (such as the wolf, dingo and coyote) in cycles involving feral animals (such as the deer, wallaby and moose).

Clinical effects

Symptoms and signs are those of slowly increasing pressure in the area of the cyst, resembling a slowly growing tumour. Although infection may be contracted in childhood, it rarely becomes apparent before adolescence, except for cysts in the brain or orbit.

In the liver, cysts grow around 1mm per month and are palpable when they approach 20cm in diameter (Fig. 2.50). Compression of the liver may result in jaundice and portal hypertension. Cholangitis may follow rupture of a cyst which can also cause anaphylactic reaction. Cysts in the lung (about 20–30 per cent of total cases) can cause coughing up

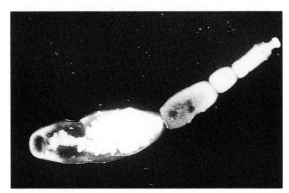

Fig. 2.49 Adult of *E. granulosus* from intestine of dog. The whole tapeworm has only 4 proglottids and measures 5mm in length.

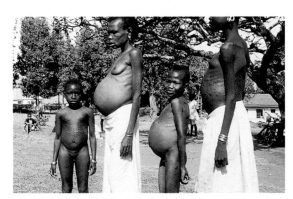

Fig. 2.50 Patients in North Kenya waiting for surgery for hydatid cysts. Courtesy of G S Nelson.

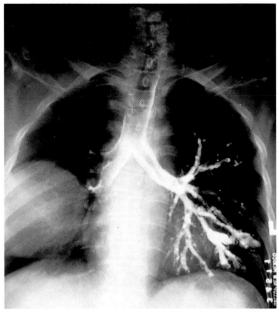

Fig. 2.51 Bronchogram (X-radiograph) of patient from Arizona showing blockage of bronchus from cyst of *E. granulosus* in lower left medial region. Courtesy of R B Holliman.

of blood (haemoptysis), difficulty in breathing (dyspnoea) and chest pain (Fig. 2.51).

About three per cent of cysts occur in the brain or spinal cord, provoking an acute inflammatory response, usually in the white matter. When this subsides, cysts become encapsulated but continue to grow slowly and cause pressure effects. Osseous cysts represent about 1–2 per cent of the total and they grow slowly, with no host reaction; sometimes cancellous bones are destroyed and collapse without warning.

Diagnosis

Clinical symptoms of a slow-growing tumour accompanied by eosinophilia are suggestive. Occasionally, lung cysts burst and hooks may be found in the sputum. Computerized axial tomography (CAT) scans (Fig. 2.52) and, to a lesser extent, X-rays can show up the hollow cysts. Portable ultrasound machines have proved helpful diagnostic aids in Kenya. An intradermal reaction (Casoni test), using hydatid fluid as antigen, is useful for epidemiological surveys (Fig. 2.53). ELISA and indirect haemagglutination have high specificity and a latex agglutination test is simple to use.

Treatment

Surgical removal of cysts is the only established form of treatment, provided that they are in a favourable site. The cyst cavity should first be sterilized with five per cent cetrimide as there is great danger from rupturing a cyst and spreading protoscoleces to new sites to form more cysts.

Mebendazole, given daily by mouth for many months, has sometimes shown promising results but often does not penetrate the thick walled cysts: albendazole looks more hopeful. Either might be particularly useful after surgery to prevent other small cysts from growing.

Prevention and control

Personal hygiene in relation to contact with dogs is important to prevent ingestion of eggs. Regular treatment campaigns against adult tapeworms in dogs with praziquantel and sanitary disposal of offal and viscera of slaughtered food animals are the most important control measures.

Causative organism	Disease
Echinococcus multilocularis	Alveolar echinococcosis

Transmission and epidemiology

Infection by *Echinococcus multilocularis* in animals is mainly holarctic, the adult tapeworms parasitizing wild carnivores such as the red and arctic foxes, while the usual intermediate hosts are the field mouse in Europe and the vole and lemming in Siberia and North America (Fig. 2.47).

The adult tapeworms are similar to *Echinococcus granulosus* but about half the size. Eggs passed in the faeces of foxes are very resistant to cold. Most

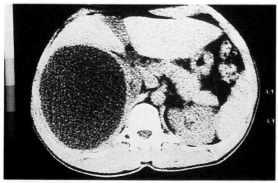

Fig. 2.52 Computerized tomography (CT) scan showing presence of large cyst of *E. granulosus* in the liver. Courtesy of A Bryceson.

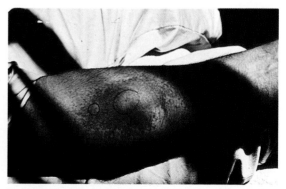

Fig. 2.53 A positive intradermal (Casoni) test using cyst fluid antigen. Serological tests are now used more often.

human cases are in fur trappers but infection can also be contracted from wild fruits, berries or vegetables contaminated with fox faeces. *E. oligarthrus* has been reported from Panama and Brazil with a life cycle involving the puma and possibly the agouti, and adults of *E. vogeli* have been recovered from a bush dog in Ecuador.

Clinical effects

Symptoms in man resemble those of a slow malignant growth, almost always in the liver (Fig. 2.54): they may take many years to develop, by which time the disease is inoperable. The thin-walled, multilocular cysts form pseudo-malignant growths with a spongy mass of proliferating vesicles embedded in a dense fibrous sheath. The cysts in man do not contain protoscoleces. There is necrosis of the surrounding liver tissue with an obliterative endarteritis. Ascites may follow portal hypertension.

Diagnosis

Early diagnosis is important: ELISA, indirect haemagglutination or latex agglutination tests can be used. CAT scans or X-rays are not so satisfactory as with *E. granulosus*.

Treatment

There is usually no appropriate treatment, although surgery can be tried in early cases. There is a tendency for cysts to bud off and spread to lymph glands, lungs, brain and other areas. Mebendazole, albendazole or praziquantel might be more effective than against the thicker-walled cysts of *E. granulosus* but have not been properly evaluated.

Prevention and control

Fur trappers should be aware of the dangers of contamination when skinning foxes.

OTHER LARVAL CESTODES

Causative organism	Disease
Taenia multiceps	Coenurus infection
(*Multiceps multiceps*)	

The adult tapeworm is a parasite of dogs and wild canids and the natural intermediate host is the sheep, or sometimes other ruminants, in which the bladder worm stage, known as a coenurus (or popularly as a gidworm causing the staggers), develops. The coenurus measures a few centimetres in diameter and differs from a cysticercus in having about 100 protoscolices projecting internally from the wall.

In most human cases from temperate areas, the coenurus has been in the brain, but in tropical areas

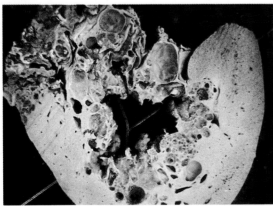

Fig. 2.54 Liver from a fatal case in man with numerous multilocular cysts of *E. multilocularis* (or possibly *E. oligarthrus*). Courtesy of Prof. R B Holliman.

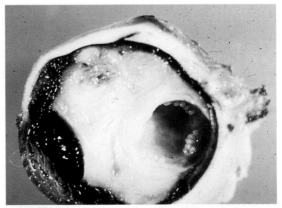

Fig. 2.55 Coenurus cyst in the vitreous chamber of a human eye. It is a simple cyst containing many protoscolices, each of which can develop into an adult *Taenia multiceps* in the dog. The usual intermediate hosts are sheep and other herbivores. Courtesy of Dr A C Templeton.

the cyst is usually subcutaneous or in the eye (Fig. 2.55). Other species may be involved in different parts of the world. In the brain, most cysts are in the subarachnoid space and give rise to a leptomeningitis with symptoms of headache and vomiting. Paralysis may result. There have been less than 100 cases reported from man, either from ingesting eggs on vegetables or from contact with dogs. It is difficult to differentiate coenurus infections from cysticercosis or echinococcosis, except after removal of cysts at surgery. Treatment with praziquantel would be effective.

Causative organism	Disease
Spirometra species	Sparganosis

Occasional cases of human infection with plerocercoid larvae (spargana) of diphyllobothriid tapeworms of the genus *Spirometra* (sometimes synonymized with *Diphyllobothrium*) have been reported. The adult tapeworms are parasites of carnivores in many parts of the world (but not of man) and procercoid larvae are found in *Cyclops* inhabiting small ponds, with plerocercoids normally in amphibia, reptiles or small mammals, or large game animals in East Africa.

Infection is usually contracted from ingesting *Cyclops* containing procercoids in drinking water, but in Thailand and Vietnam infection may be by applying split amphibia containing plerocercoids to sores and infected eyes. Spargana wander in the deep tissues and usually migrate to the subcutaneous tissues (Fig. 2.56), eliciting a local inflammatory response and eventually encysting; the result is a fibrous nodule, about 2cm in diameter. Ocular sparganosis causes intense pain with periportal oedema and ulceration. Praziquantel might be effective.

NEMATODES

Nematodes, popularly known as roundworms, are one of the most widespread and successful group of animals, colonizing a wide range of habitats including most parts of the human body. They are typically cylindrical, tapering at each end. Those parasitic in man may be large stout worms such as *Ascaris*, minute microscopic forms such as *Strongyloides*, or long, threadlike organisms such as the filariae.

The body is covered with a thick, colourless, acellular cuticle, containing numerous diagonally arranged collagen fibres which allow some alteration

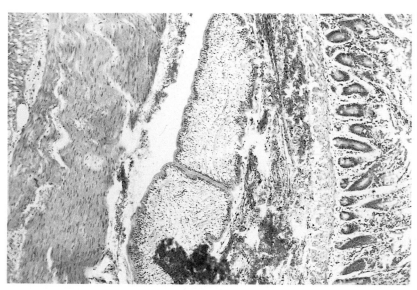

Fig. 2.56 Section of the wall of the small intestine (of monkey) with migrating plerocercoid (sparganum) of *Spirometra*, causing disruption and haemorrhage.

in body length. The sexes are separate and morphologically distinct, the male usually having copulatory spicules at the tail end, and sometimes also an enlargement of the tail known as a caudal bursa. All forms have a complete gut with both mouth and anus; the mouth sometimes leading into an enlarged buccal capsule, perhaps containing cuticularized structures for cutting into tissues (Fig. 2.57).

During the life cycle, there are a series of four moults when the cuticle is shed and, in most parasites of man, the third larval stage is responsible for infecting a new host.

About 14 species of nematodes are principally parasites of man, while about 50 others can attack the human body, although more usually found in animals.

Some of the human nematode infections are widespread: *Ascaris*, for example occurs in about 22 per cent of the world population (one billion people) and the lymphatic filariae in about 7 per cent.

The nematodes of man can be divided into two groups: the intestinal nematodes with a direct life cycle in which eggs or larvae in the environment or on salad vegetables are infective to a new host (such as the roundworms, hookworms, whipworms, *Strongyloides* and pinworms); tissue nematodes with an indirect life cycle involving an intermediate host which can be an arthropod (filariae and guinea

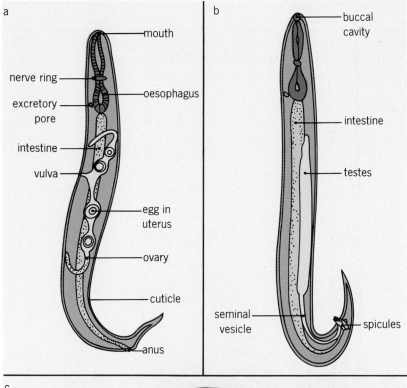

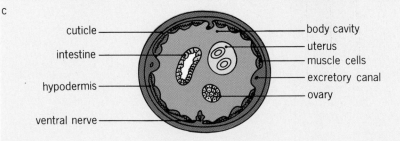

Fig. 2.57 Diagrams showing the principal features of adult nematodes (based on *Strongyloides*). (a) Female (parasitic); (b) Male (free-living); (c) Cross section (of female).

worms) or another vertebrate (trichina worms). Those intestinal nematodes which require a period in the soil for larval development are known as 'geo–helminths'.

INTESTINAL NEMATODES

Intestinal nematode eggs are illustrated in Fig. 2.58 and their sizes given in Fig. 2.59.

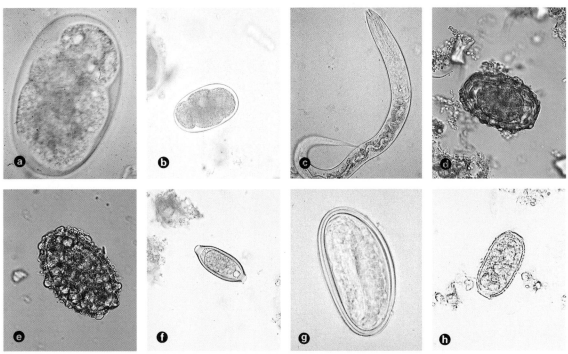

Fig. 2.58 Eggs and larvae of intestinal nematodes passed in faeces. (a) Egg of *Necator americanus* or *Ancylostoma duodenale* (identical). (b) Egg of hookworm under low power. Note that ovum continues to divide and may be at 16- or 32- celled stage in old faecal sample. (c) Larva of *Strongyloides*
stercoralis. (d) Egg of *Ascaris* (fertile). (e) Egg of *Ascaris* (infertile: about 15 per cent are like this). (f) Egg of *Trichuris*. (g) Egg of *Enterobius* (on perianal skin rather than in faeces). (h) Egg of *Capillaria philippinensis*. Courtesy of J H Cross.

Fig. 2.59 Sizes of intestinal nematode eggs.

Species	Size of egg
Necator americanus Ancylostoma duodenale	60 × 50μm
Strongyloides stercoralis	250μm (larva)
Ascaris	60 × 40μm
Trichuris	50 × 20μm
Enterobius	55 × 25μm
Capillaria philippinensis	40 × 21μm

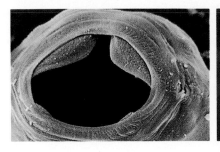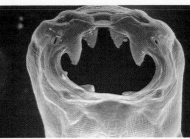

Fig. 2.60 Scanning electron micrographs of the anterior ends of adult *Necator* (left) and *Ancyclostoma* (right), showing the cutting plates in the mouth of the former and 'teeth' in the latter for biting off pieces of mucosa. Courtesy of Dr L M Gibbons.

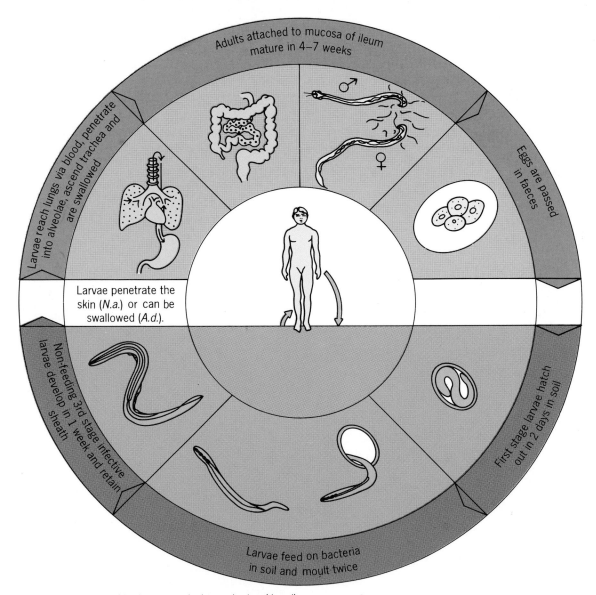

Adults attached to mucosa of ileum mature in 4–7 weeks

Larvae reach lungs via blood, penetrate into alveolae, ascend trachea and are swallowed

Eggs are passed in faeces

Larvae penetrate the skin (*N.a.*) or can be swallowed (*A.d.*).

Non-feeding 3rd stage infective larvae develop in 1 week and retain sheath

First stage larvae hatch out in 2 days in soil

Larvae feed on bacteria in soil and moult twice

Fig. 2.61 Life cycle of hookworms in the human host and in soil.

Causative organism	Disease
Necator americanus	New World hookworm disease
Ancylostoma	Old World hookworm disease
	Both cause hookworm anaemia

Transmission and epidemiology

Adult hookworms live in the jejunum with the anterior end attached to the mucosa. Morphologically, they have a sharply bent back head and a large buccal capsule (Fig. 2.60); males have an expanded caudal bursa. Females of *Ancylostoma* measure 12 × 0.6 mm and males 10 × 0.4 mm; *Necator* is slightly smaller.

The life cycle is illustrated in Fig. 2.61. Oval, thin-shelled eggs are passed in the faeces and are usually at the four-celled stage of development (see Fig. 2.58).

When the eggs reach moist soil the larvae develop and hatch out in approximately 24 hours. Larvae feed in the soil, moult twice, and reach the infective third stage in five days. The third-stage larvae do not feed and they retain the larval sheath, requiring warmth, shade and moisture and preferring a light sandy soil. They can live in the soil for a few weeks but must penetrate the skin of a new host (although *Ancylostoma* larvae may be swallowed on raw vegetables, when larvae penetrate through the mucosa of the mouth) in order to develop further.

Hookworm infection is limited mainly to tropical and subtropical regions (Fig. 2.62) because the larvae cannot develop below 22°C and is most common in rural areas with an annual rainfall of over 100 cm per year. *Ancylostoma* larvae can survive at lower temperatures than those of *Necator* and were found in mines and among tunnel builders in Europe. It is estimated that there are around 800 million cases in the world, with 1.6 million suffering from anaemia and 55 000 deaths annually.

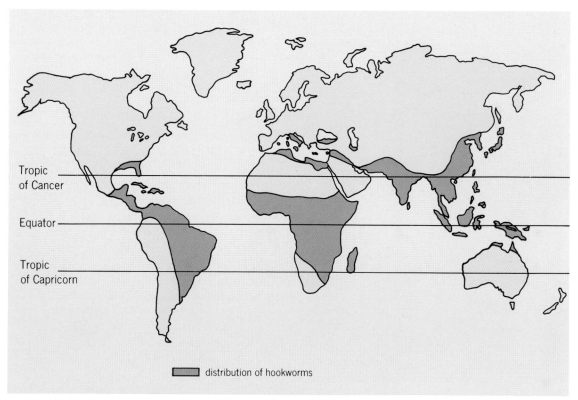

Fig. 2.62 Distribution map of human hookworms (*Necator* and *Ancylostoma*).

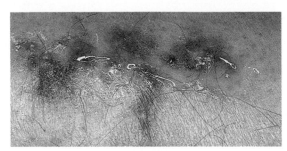

Fig. 2.63 Dermatitis in sensitized individual caused by penetraton of *Necator* larvae ('ground itch').

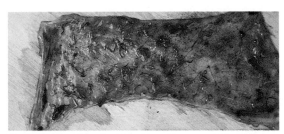

Fig. 2.64 A portion of cat intestine with many adult hookworms causing extensive haemorrhagic patches. The gut of each worm is filled with blood.

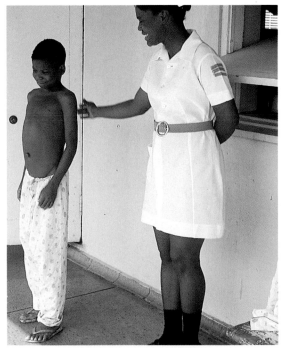

Fig. 2.65 Youth of 17 with very heavy chronic hookworm infection, anaemia, and severe stunting of growth (height 1.35m).

Larvae of dog hookworms can sometimes penetrate human skin but do not develop further. They form serpentine, inflammatory channels under the skin, the condition known as cutaneous larva migrans or creeping eruption.

Clinical effects

A few days after penetration of the larvae, a local dermatitis, known as ground itch, develops (Fig. 2.63); after repeated reinfection this may be severe with blisters and papular eruptions. Two to four weeks after infection, pneumonitis develops, caused by the migrating larvae in the lungs.

With light infections there are few or no gastro-intestinal symptoms but in heavier infections there are likely to be epigastric pains.

Hookworms are blood feeders, so the most serious consequence of heavy infection is an iron deficiency anaemia. Hookworms bite off pieces of mucosa (Fig. 2.64) and pass blood through their bodies for both nutrition and respiration. They change their attachment site often, so that in heavy infections 100ml of blood may be lost per day (about 0.15ml for each adult *Ancylostoma*).

In endemic areas, high worm loads are sometimes associated with retardation of growth in children (Fig. 2.65) and severe anaemia with ensuing cardiac symptoms and oedema.

Diagnosis

Chronic anaemia and debility are suggestive but need parasitological confirmation. The characteristic eggs (see Figs 2.58 & 2.59) can be recognized in stool samples examined by light microscopy. Concentration methods can be used if eggs are scarce. The eggs of the two species are identical; a smear of faeces on moist filter paper in a closed tube can be kept for a few days in order to differentiate the larvae which hatch out and develop (see p.137).

Haemagglutination and complement fixation tests can be employed for immunodiagnosis but have not been widely used.

Treatment

New wide-spectrum anthelmintics have revolutionized the treatment of all geohelminth infections. These drugs include albendazole, mebendazole, levamisole and pyrantel pamoate. Older more specific drugs, such as bephenium and tetrachlorethylene, are still employed because they are much cheaper.

Iron therapy for the anaemia is a very important supplement to any anthelmintic.

Prevention and control
Personal protection is provided by wearing shoes (larvae usually penetrate through the feet) and, for *Ancylostoma*, washing of salad vegetables.

Control principally involves an increase in sanitary conditions, coupled with regular chemotherapeutic campaigns; such an approach has reduced infection rates from 25 per cent to almost nil in Japan in the last 40 years.

Causative organism	Disease
Strongyloides stercoralis	Strongyloidiasis

Transmission and epidemiology
The life cycle is illustrated in Fig. 2.66. The minute (2.0mm long) adult parthenogenetic females live

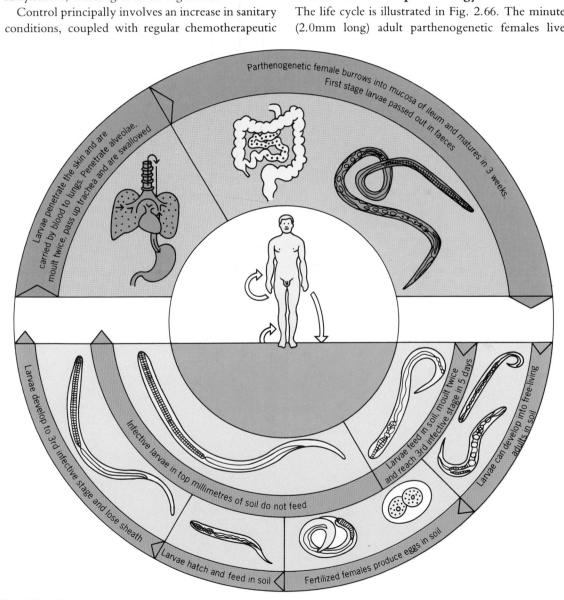

Fig. 2.66 Life cycle of *Strongyloides stercoralis*.

embedded in the mucosa of the small intestine (Fig. 2.67). They produce eggs, which hatch in the intestine into first-stage (rhabditiform) larvae measuring 0.25mm. Larvae are passed out in faeces and feed on bacteria in the soil. After a few days they have moulted twice; the infective third-stage (filariform) larvae can live in soil for around 12 days but once they are in contact with the skin of a new host they penetrate it. Inside the body the development is similar to that of hookworms. Sometimes, however, larvae in the soil develop into either females or males which undergo one or more free-living cycles in the soil before producing infective larvae again.

Self infection can occur if larvae have developed to the infective stage by the time they reach the anus and then penetrate through the perianal skin. In this way infection can persist for many years after an individual has left an endemic area, even though adult females live for only a few months. Such infections typically show recurrent skin rashes (larva currens) caused by the fast moving larvae (5–10mm per hour) and are still found in ex-prisoners of war over 40 years after leaving an endemic area.

S. stercoralis is a cosmopolitan parasite with a similar distribution to the hookworms (see Fig. 2.62) and is particularly important in South America and SE Asia; the larvae need similar conditions of a warm, moist, light soil thus confining infection to the tropics and subtropics, particularly where sanitary standards are low.

Another species, *S. fuelleborni*, in which eggs rather than larvae are passed out in faeces, is a common parasite of primates in Africa and Asia and is often found in man in Central Africa. The same or a similar form is the cause of a very virulent disease of infants in Papua New Guinea.

Clinical effects

The majority of infected people appear to suffer no ill effect, although there is likely to be an itchy rash a few days after infection, followed by mild respiratory symptoms in a few weeks.

Severe infection is rare but manifestations include vomiting, severe abdominal pain, abdominal distension, diarrhoea with voluminous stools and a malabsorption syndrome with dehydration and electrolyte disturbance. In such cases larvae penetrate the submucosa; the mucosa becomes flattened and atrophies and there is a marked loss of elasticity of the intestinal wall. Abdominal lymph nodes are also enlarged.

In the majority of individuals who are lightly infected there are no apparent symptoms. In heavy infections, dysentery, anorexia, nausea, abdominal pain and weight loss with finger clubbing are apparent. Very heavy infections in poorly nourished individuals can produce anaemia from the blood loss.

In some situations, particularly in immunocompromised patients undergoing cancer therapy or with AIDS, first-stage larvae may develop into the infective forms, penetrate the intestinal wall and then invade lymph nodes and other organs (hyperinfection). Hyperinfection is probably usually fatal and can appear years after first infection.

Diagnosis

Clinically, a watery diarrhoea with mucus and eosinophilia, accompanied by a larval rash in the anal region, are characteristic. Larva currens lasting a few hours may appear on the buttocks, groin or lower trunk for a few days every few weeks. Radiological pictures of the lower duodenum after a barium meal are likely to show abnormalities in clinical cases.

Larvae (measuring 0.25mm) in the faeces provide a positive diagnosis. If they are scarce, concentration techniques can be used. Alternatively, examination of a swallowed brushed nylon string in a gelatin capsule may reveal first-stage larvae, or a faecal sample can be cultured on moist filter paper strips for a few days and examined for infective larvae.

Immunodiagnostic methods, such as indirect

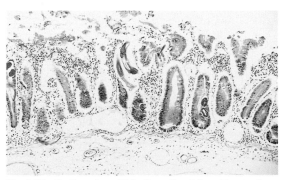

Fig. 2.67 Section of small intestine with adult and larvae of *Strongyloides stercoralis* in the mucosa. Note disruption of villous surface.

haemagglutination and complement fixation, are sensitive but not very specific.

Treatment

Of the newer drugs, albendazole has some action; thiabendazole has been widely used in recent years although it has unpleasant side effects. It is not certain if either of these compounds provides a permanent cure in clinical cases and neither is effective in cases of disseminated strongyloidiasis (hyper-infection). Levamisole will also kill adult worms.

Any anthelmintic treatment should be repeated after a few weeks.

Prevention and control

The wearing of shoes will go a long way toward preventing infection. Control requires sanitary disposal of faeces and possibly mass chemotherapy, which can only be envisaged as part of a campaign against geohelminths in general.

Causative organism	Disease
Ascaris lumbricoides	Roundworm infection Ascariasis

Transmission and epidemiology

Adults are large, thick, white worms, females measuring 300 × 8mm and males 200 × 5mm.

The life cycle is illustrated in Fig. 2.68. Infection is contracted by ingesting embryonated eggs (see Fig. 2.58) on salad vegetables or, with young children, in

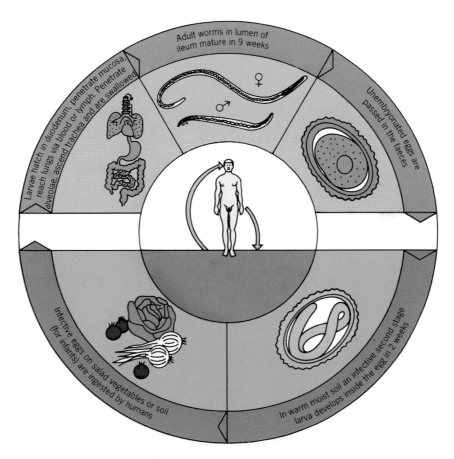

Fig. 2.68 Life cycle of *Ascaris lumbricoides*.

soil. The second stage larvae inside eggs hatch in the duodenum and penetrate the wall to reach the bloodstream, whence they are carried to the lungs. In the lungs the larvae grow and moult (twice) before penetrating the alveolae and returning to the intestine, via the trachea and oesophagus. In the ileum they mature into males and females and mate; the females produce about 200 000 eggs per day, commencing about 65 days after infection. Adults live free in the lumen of the gut for 6 months to 2 years. Eggs, thick-shelled and very resistant to sewage digestion, high temperatures (up to 45°C) and drying (down to 6 per cent), are passed in the faeces and the larvae inside develop quickly in warm moist soil, particularly clay, or water (10 days at 30°C; 50 days at 17°C).

Infection is very common, particularly in children, in most tropical and subtropical countries (and in temperate regions with a warm summer) where there is high rainfall (Fig. 2.69). About three quarters of all cases are in Southeast Asia. There are estimated to be one billion (1000m) infections worldwide.

Clinical effects

The larvae in the lungs can cause pneumonitis, with a cough, chest pain and difficulty in breathing (Löffler's syndrome); a pronounced pulmonary eosinophilia may occur.

In the majority of infected persons, the few adult worms present (mean number is 6) result in minor symptoms or none. It is estimated, however, that worldwide, *Ascaris* causes one million cases of clinical disease with 20 000 deaths annually. Even a small worm load can cause allergic reactions in sensitized individuals.

Large numbers of worms (over 100) can result in digestive disorders and, particularly in children,

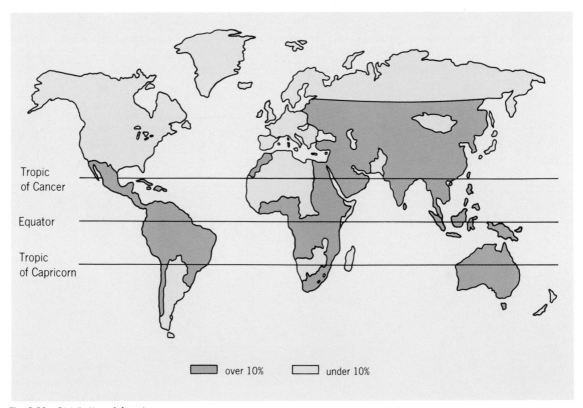

Fig. 2.69 Distribution of *Ascaris*.

protein energy malnutrition. Intestinal obstruction (Fig. 2.70) results in symptoms of severe abdominal pain, nausea and vomiting; worms in the bile duct lead to severe colicky pains and cholangitis. *Ascaris* are easily irritated and can wander out through the mouth or nose or become embedded in abdominal stitches.

Diagnosis

Unembryonated eggs are usually present in large numbers in the faeces. They have a thick, mamillated, albuminous outer coat. If necessary, concentration by sedimentation can be employed. Adult *Ascaris* can often be diagnosed as a filling defect in straight X-rays of the abdomen (Fig. 2.71) and intravenous cholangiography can help in cases of biliary obstruction.

Treatment

New drugs used against hookworms, such as albendazole, mebendazole (although this sometimes causes worms to wander), levamisole and pyrantel pamoate are also effective against *Ascaris*. Piperazine has been used for the last 40 years and is very successful and cheap; its main disadvantage is that it does not have a very broad spectrum of activity.

Cases of bile duct or intestinal obstruction should be treated conservatively with intravenous fluids but without surgery if possible.

Prevention and control

Thorough washing of salad vegetables is necessary for personal protection.

Improvement in sanitary conditions and disposal of excreta, coupled with regular chemotherapy, can reduce intensity and, probably, prevalence of infection in time. However, a few heavily infected individuals can pass a high proportion of all eggs produced to maintain transmission; such cases should be targets for chemotherapy.

Causative organism	Disease
Trichuris trichiura	Trichuriasis; whipworm infection

Transmission and epidemiology

The adults of both sexes have a narrow anterior portion and wider posterior end and measure about 40mm. The male has a tightly coiled tail.

Infection is contracted from ingesting embryonated eggs on salad vegetables or, in young children, in soil. The contained first-stage larva hatches in the

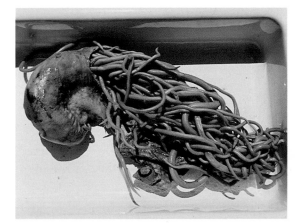

Fig. 2.70 Portion of small intestine completely blocked by *Ascaris*. Courtesy of Prof. R B Holliman.

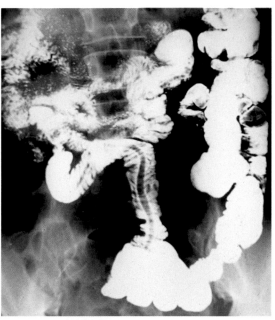

Fig. 2.71 X-ray after barium meal with filling defect in small intestine showing presence of adult *Ascaris*. Courtesy of Prof. W Peters.

intestine and grows to adulthood in the caecum. The adults live with their anterior ends embedded in the mucosa (Fig. 2.72). After mating, females produce eggs in 2–3 months and normally live for about 3 years. Each female produces around 10 000 eggs per day which are passed in the faeces. At tropical temperatures on soil a larva develops quickly inside the egg (17 days at 30°C compared to 4 months at 15°C).

Trichuris is found in the same areas in which *Ascaris* is prevalent (p.98) with around 800 million cases in the world.

Clinical effects

In children there may be retarded growth and malnutrition, occasionally with prolapse of the rectum (Fig. 2.73).

Pathologically, the worms cause inflammation of the caecum and colon, and in heavy infections, the lower ileum and rectum.

Diagnosis

This is made by finding the easily recognized eggs in the faeces, using concentration techniques if necessary. Sometimes adults can be seen hanging from the colon wall by using a sigmoidoscope.

Treatment

Because of the inaccessible site of the adults treatment is difficult. Albendazole and mebendazole have some action, as does oxantel in a mixture with pyrantel pamoate. Thiabendazole was until recently the only effective treatment but it has unpleasant side effects.

Prevention and control

Prevention involves thorough washing of salad vegetables. Control is by improvement in sanitary conditions coupled with regular deworming campaigns: a slow business.

Causative organism	Disease
Enterobius vermicularis	pinworm, threadworm or seatworm infection

Transmission and epidemiology

Pinworms are small cylindrical nematodes (female 11 × 0.4mm, males 3 × 0.2mm). A gravid female migrates out of the anus at night and lays numerous sticky eggs on the anal skin. Sometimes she bursts and releases all the eggs (which number about 10 000), and this can cause intense itching. Eggs on the skin develop to an infective stage in a few hours at body temperature and may also be carried in house dust.

Enterobius is one of the most common of all parasitic infections in the world and is often a group infection, particularly common in children and in institutions in temperate climates. Its spread is contaminative rather than soil-transmitted, often from the anus to the hand of an infected individual to the hand and then the mouth of another person.

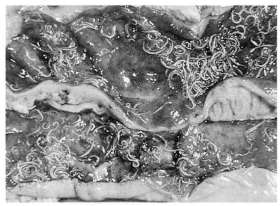

Fig. 2.72 Colon opened to show many adult *Trichuris*. The thinner anterior end of each worm is embedded in the mucosa, causing haemorrhagic patches. Courtesy of Prof. R B Holliman.

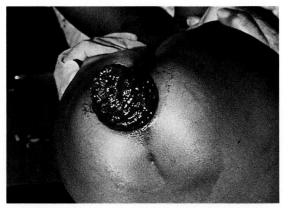

Fig. 2.73 Young child with prolapsed rectum, showing some adult *Trichuris*. They cause irritation and hyperaemia which results in straining. Courtesy of Dr H Zaiman.

Clinical effects

Infection is often symptomless or with anal itching (*pruritis ani*) caused by a reaction to the sticky eggs; this can result in disturbed sleep in children and secondary bacterial infection consequent on scratching. In a few cases there may be mild catarrhal inflammation with diarrhoea and slight eosinophilia. Appendicitis has been reported from worms blocking the appendix and in girls vaginitis is not uncommon.

Diagnosis

Ova are rarely found in the faeces and are usually looked for by wiping the anal region with sticky tape first thing in the morning and sticking this onto a microscope slide for examination. Repeated examinations may be necessary but are not really warranted for such a minor infection. Adult worms are often observed on the surface of stools.

Treatment

Albendazole and mebendazole are both very effective as are levamisole and pyrantel pamoate. Piperazine has been effectively used for the last 40 years but requires a course of treatment over a few days. Whichever compound is used it is advisable to treat the entire family or group.

Prevention and control

Following chemotherapy hygienic measures are very important, with frequent washing of hands and bedclothes and cleaning of rooms. The eggs can survive for many days in moist, cool, house dust and for a few days on toys or furniture.

Causative organism	Disease
Capillaria philippinensis	intestinal capillariasis

Transmission and epidemiology

This is a recently discovered parasite reported from Luzon, Philippines, with a few cases in Thailand and Iran. Adults measure 3mm and burrow into the mucosa of the small intestine. Freshwater fish, eaten raw or undercooked, appear to act as intermediate hosts. Eggs passed in the faeces of the natural hosts (birds perhaps) presumably embryonate in water, are ingested by fish and larvae develop in their muscles.

Clinical effects

Intermittent diarrhoea with characteristic 'tummy gurgles' and abdominal pain. Symptoms resemble tropical sprue with many and voluminous stools and malabsorption. Muscle wasting, emaciation and weakness occur in many patients, and mortality of untreated cases is over 20 per cent, principally from heart failure.

This is an unusual nematode infection as it appears that the parasites can multiply in the intestine when larvae hatch from eggs in the body. The adults and larvae become embedded in the ileum wall, causing flattening of the villi.

Diagnosis

Eggs can be found in the faeces and are somewhat similar to those of *Trichuris* (Fig. 2.58).

Treatment

Thiabendazole has a dramatic effect but relapses may occur; mebendazole has now replaced it.

Protection and control

Cooking of freshwater fish which appear to be the intermediate hosts should provide personal protection. Man is not a natural host and there is unlikely to be person to person transmission.

Causative organism	Disease
Ternidens deminutus	False hookworm infection

Ternidens inhabits the colon and occasionally the ileum of man in Central and South Africa. Adults suck blood but infections are almost always light and symptomless. Eggs in the faeces are very similar to those of hookworm and treatment is identical. The mode of transmission is unknown.

Causative organism	Disease
Anisakis spp.	Herringworm disease
Pseudoterranova decipiens	Codworm disease

Anisakis and *Pseudoterranova* are natural parasites of marine fish-eating mammals; human cases occur where the intermediate host marine fish are eaten raw (for example, Japan and the Netherlands). In man the larvae cause abscesses in the stomach or intestinal wall. Most cases are diagnosed in tissue sections of biopsy specimens. Deep freezing of fish prevents infection.

TISSUE NEMATODES

This disparate group of nematodes all have an indirect life-cycle involving more than one host. Some are natural parasites of man, such as the filariae

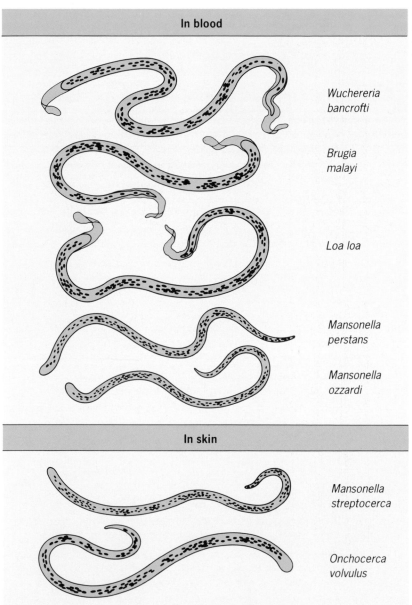

In blood

Wuchereria bancrofti

Brugia malayi

Loa loa

Mansonella perstans

Mansonella ozzardi

In skin

Mansonella streptocerca

Onchocerca volvulus

Fig. 2.74 Microfilariae: comparison of species. Important diagnostic differences are related to the presence or absence of a sheath, relative size and the structure of the tail region.

which have insects as intermediate hosts, and the guinea worm which utilizes water fleas (cyclops); others are only accidental parasites of man, such as the trichina worms in which larvae are transmitted in the flesh of many mammals.

Adult filariae (superfamily Filarioidea) are all long, thin, string-like nematodes, some of which are responsible for important human diseases. The females are all viviparous, producing early first-stage larvae known as microfilariae, rather than eggs, and these are released into the bloodstream or tissue spaces for ingestion by an insect vector. Microfilariae measure 150–350μm in length and specific identification is important in diagnosis; in some filariae, such as *Wuchereria*, *Brugia* and *Loa*, microfilariae retain the shell of the egg to form a sheath, while in others, such as *Onchocerca* and *Mansonella*, the shell is lost and they are unsheathed (Fig. 2.74).

Causative organism	Disease
Wuchereria; Brugia	lymphatic filariasis
Wuchereria bancrofti	bancroftian filariasis
Brugia malayi	malayan filariasis
Brugia timori	timorian filariasis

Transmission and epidemiology

The adults (females measuring 80–100mm × 0.25mm, males 40mm × 0.1mm) live in the lymphatic glands and lymph vessels of either the lower limbs and groin or, in the case of *Wuchereria*, the upper limbs also.

Sheathed microfilariae reach the blood and travel around the bloodstream at night, while during the day they hide in the lung capillaries (nocturnal periodicity). In the eastern Pacific (Fig. 2.75) the vectors are day-biting mosquitoes so that microfilariae are found also during the day (subperiodic).

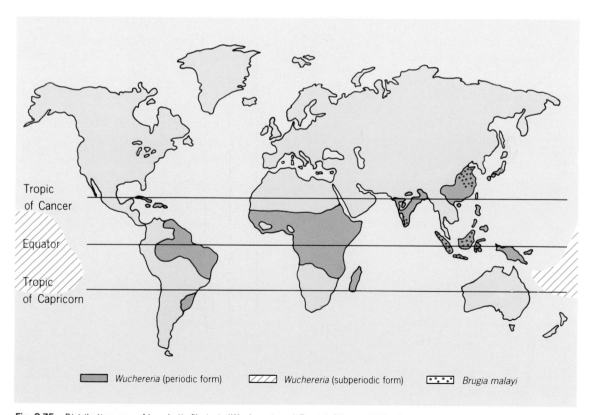

Fig. 2.75 Distribution map of lymphatic filariasis (*Wuchereria* and *Brugia*). Of around 90 million cases in the world 60 per cent are in China, India and Indonesia.

To develop further the microfilariae must be picked up by a mosquito in a blood meal as depicted in the life cycle diagram (Fig. 2.76). There are two moults in the mosquito: the infective third-stage larvae penetrate the proboscis sheath and enter the lymphatics through the puncture wound. Infective third-stage larvae measure 1.6mm.

Various mosquitoes breed in old tin cans, latrines

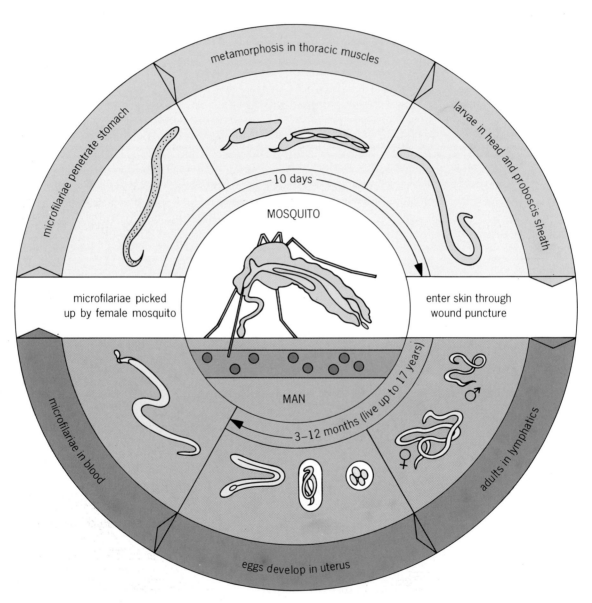

Fig. 2.76   Life cycle of lymphatic filariae.

or ponds. The most important species worldwide for *Wuchereria* is the 'urban' *quinquefasciatus* (see Chapter 3 p.120). However, depending on the region, the mosquito vector may be one or two of around eighty species of *Anopheles*, *Culex*, *Aedes* and *Mansonia*.

W. bancrofti is found only in man but a subperiodic form of *B. malayi* is maintained also in forest monkeys, and possibly cats in Thailand, Malaysia, Indonesia and the Philippines, and principally affects man in rice-growing areas close to forest.

Clinical effects

There are often no symptoms initially and in some cases none appear. Usually, the first clinical manifestations develop 8–16 months after infection, although they may be delayed for much longer in individuals raised in an endemic area, or accelerated in immigrants. Acute manifestations consist of a recurrent adenolymphangitis (inflammation of the lymph ducts), particularly in the groin region, with episodes of fever, nausea, headaches and possibly a rash ('filarial fever') lasting up to two weeks. The symptoms appear at regular intervals and are usually accompanied by eosinophilia (an increase in the numbers of circulating eosinophils). Sometimes there is lymphadenitis (inflammation of the lymph nodes, Fig. 2.77) and in males, orchitis and funiculitis (inflammation of the spermatic cords).

Adults of nocturnally periodic *W. bancrofti* and *Brugia* usually develop in the lymphatics of the lower limbs, while those of the subperiodic Pacific strain of *W. bancrofti* are also found in the lymphatics of the upper limbs.

In bancroftian filariasis, adult worms often block the spermatic lymph vessels; as the scrotal sac becomes distended with lymph, hydrocoele and chyluria (lymph appearing in the urine) result (Fig. 2.78).

In timorian filariasis, abscesses and secondary bacterial infections of the lymph vessels, and ulcers on the legs along the track of the swollen lymphatics are particularly common.

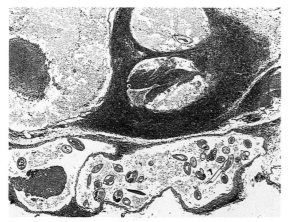

Fig. 2.77 Transverse section of a lymph node at an early clinical stage of infection with adult *Wuchereria*. It shows dilated lymphatics and tissue reaction in the walls of the vessels.

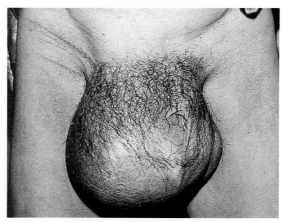

Fig. 2.78 Hydrocoele. This is the most common clinical effect of bancroftian filariasis in males in many parts of the world, particularly East Africa and the Pacific. Courtesy of Prof. W Peters; Wolfe Medical Books.

In a small proportion of cases, the oedematous lymph nodes become infiltrated by so many plasma cells, and then fibroblasts, that the channels are completely blocked and they eventually calcify (Fig. 2.79). The affected parts of the body are bathed in lymph and enlarge (lymphoedema), which eventually leads to the grotesque and disfiguring elephantiasis, with the growth of possibly several kilograms of new tissue. In *Brugia* infections, elephantiasis occurs on the lower limbs below the knee (Fig. 2.80) but in bancroftian filariasis can also affect the genitals and sometimes the arms and breasts.

The most chronic and irreversible changes may take 10–15 years to develop and elephantiasis usually only develops in adult life. Symptomatic cases of filariasis appear to be associated with immunopathological reactions of the host; patients with elephantiasis rarely have circulating microfilariae since they are rapidly destroyed. Why only some patients become sensitized in this way is unknown. A diagrammatic course of the disease is shown (Fig. 2.81).

Occasionally, tropical pulmonary eosinophilia (TPE) develops in which microfilariae are not found in the blood ('occult' filariasis). There is chest pain, cough, fever and difficulty in breathing with a very high eosinophilia (up to 35 per cent eosinophils in the blood). It can lead to chronic pulmonary fibrosis but resolves rapidly with diethylcarbamazine (DEC).

Diagnosis

Routinely this is parasitological, by identifying the characteristic sheathed microfilariae in a thick blood film taken at night from a patient's finger or ear, haemolysed, fixed and stained (Fig. 2.82). Microfilariae of *W. bancrofti* measure around 260μm, while those of *B. malayi* measure around 230μm in length.

A simple diagnostic method is to examine a drop of blood in water in a counting chamber on a microscope slide (see p.138). For very low microfilaraemias, 1–10ml of venous blood can be collected in a syringe, passed through a cellulose membrane filter (5μm pore size), and examined under a microscope.

Serological methods (IFAT and ELISA) work best in amicrofilaraemic cases which are clinically the most important and also the most difficult to diagnose parasitologically, but are not very useful for surveys.

Treatment

Chemotherapy with DEC has been used since 1947. When given every day for 2–3 weeks, it kills microfilariae effectively but is not active against adult worms; treatment may have to be repeated every few months. Recently, very low doses given continuously for several months have been more effective against adults.

Prevention and control

Houses should be sprayed with insecticide and ceilings built inside huts. Treated mosquito nets over beds and screens over windows are important for individual protection. Any small water bodies such as tin cans and coconut shells should be cleared.

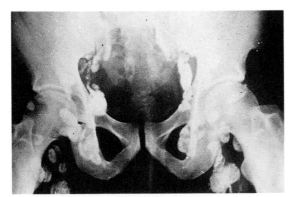

Fig. 2.79 Radiograph of chronically infected lymphatics showing calcification of the inguinal lymph nodes and ducts.

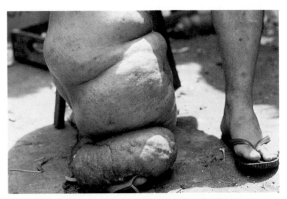

Fig. 2.80 Elephantiasis of the leg in a case of malayan filariasis. Courtesy of Dr A E Bianco.

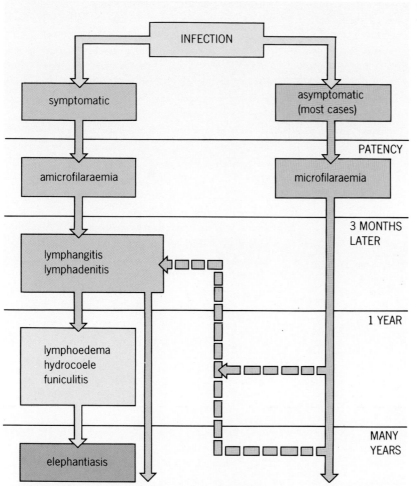

Fig. 2.81 Course of lymphatic filariasis in symptomatic cases.

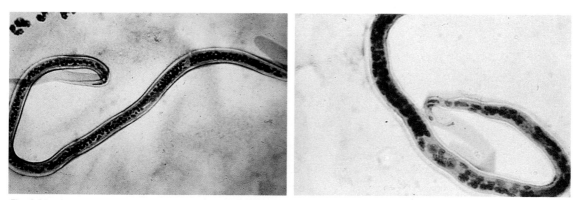

Fig. 2.82 Microfilaria of *Wuchereria bancrofti* in stained blood smear (left). It has no nuclei in the tail and is surrounded by a sheath. Microfilaria of *Brugia malayi* in blood smear (right). It has two isolated nuclei in the tail and is also surrounded by a sheath.

Non-toxic insecticides can be added to drinking water pots and larger water bodies sprayed.

Latrines are particularly important for *Culex* breeding and should have a trap to prevent the escape of adult mosquitoes, and can have a layer of polystyrene beads to prevent larvae breeding. Removal of water plants that are necessary for the development of larval *Mansonia* vectors of *B. malayi* has helped to markedly reduce prevalence in Sri Lanka and southern India.

Repeated mass chemotherapy with DEC has been successfully used in the Pacific, China, Malaysia, Indonesia and Japan. In some countries, it has been added to cooking salt.

Causative organism	Disease
Loa loa	Calabar swellings or loiasis
Mansonella ozzardi	ozzardi filariasis
Mansonella perstans	perstans filariasis
Mansonella streptocerca	streptocercal filariasis

Transmission and epidemiology

Microfilariae of *Loa*, measuring 250–300μm in length, travel in the peripheral bloodstream during the day and hide in the lung capillaries at night (diurnal periodicity). In order to develop further, they must be picked up by a large, tabanid fly *Chrysops* (mango-, softly-softly- or deer-fly; see Chapter 3). The microfilariae develop in the fat body, and infective third-stage larvae reach the mouthparts in 10–12 days. When a fly bites a new host, the larvae enter at the site of the wound and develop into adults (the females measure 70mm × 0.4mm) in the subcutaneous connective tissues within 6–12 months.

Loa is confined to rain forest areas of Central and West Africa (Fig. 2.83). Infections tend to be more common in cleared areas, such as rubber plantations, where the flies which live in the forest canopy can see movement below.

The unsheathed microfilariae of *Mansonella perstans* and *M. ozzardi* are present in the blood during the day as well as night (aperiodic), while those of *M.*

Fig. 2.83 Geographical distribution of *Loa* and of *M. ozzardi*, *M. perstans* and *M. streptocerca*.

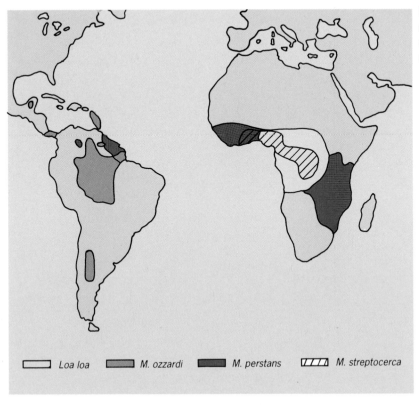

☐ *Loa loa*	▨ *M. ozzardi*	▤ *M. perstans*	▨ *M. streptocerca*

streptocerca appear in the skin. All measure about 200 × 4μm. They are transmitted by tiny biting midges, *Culicoides*, developing in the thoracic muscles and reaching the infective stage in 8 days (see Chapter 3). *M. ozzardi* occurs in Central and South America, and the West Indies; *M. perstans* in Brazil, Guyana, Surinam, as well as Central and West Africa, and *M. streptocerca* in West and Central Africa (Fig. 2.83).

Clinical effects

Adult *Loa* move through the connective tissues, causing painless, oedematous, Calabar swellings which disappear in a few days and reappear elsewhere. These swellings may be accompanied by itching, fever and generalized pruritis; there is often a high eosinophilia. Adults may also cross the conjunctiva in a matter of minutes or stay for days, causing some discomfort. High microfilariaemias can result in encephalitis, and have been associated with endomyocardial fibrosis and low fertility.

Adult *Mansonella ozzardi* and *M. perstans* live in the abdominal mesenteries and can cause manifestations such as pruritis, articular pains, headache and enlarged inguinal lymph nodes, together with eosinophilia, typical of an allergic reaction.

Adult *M. streptocerca* live in the subcutaneous connective tissue. Symptoms of infection include hypopigmented macules, oedema and thickening of skin, as well as pruritis and papules mimicking leprosy or mild onchocerciasis.

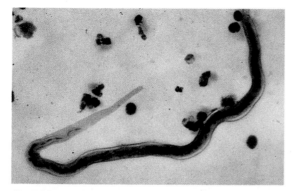

Fig. 2.84 Microfilaria of *Loa loa* in blood film taken during the day and stained with haematoxylin (Giemsa does not stain the sheath). It has nuclei to the tip of the tail.

Diagnosis

Diagnosis is parasitological, by identifying microfilariae in the blood (Fig. 2.84), or in a snip of skin in the case of *M. streptocerca*. Many patients with loiasis, however, have no circulating microfilariae (amicrofilaraemic or 'occult' infections).

Treatment

DEC kills microfilariae of *Loa* and *M. streptocerca*, but has only a slow action against adults. Meningo-encephalitis has followed treatment of cases of *Loa* with high microfilaraemias, however, and the drug should be given in a low dose initially and the effects monitored.

Prevention and control

No effective control measures exist in endemic areas, although vectors of *M. perstans* often breed in rotting banana stumps and these can be cleared. A possible preventive measure would be regular prophylactic chemotherapy with DEC.

Causative organism	Disease
Onchocerca volvulus	Onchocerciasis
	River blindness
	'Sowda'

Transmission and epidemiology

For further development, the microfilariae in the skin must be picked up by a biting blackfly, *Simulium*, which is a pool-feeder on tissue fluids. Inside the fly, the microfilariae penetrate the gut to reach the flight muscles, and there they moult twice; next, they migrate to the head and develop into infective third-stage larvae in about one week. When the fly bites a new host, the larvae enter the puncture wound, migrate to the subcutaneous tissues, and develop into adult males and females in around 12 months (the females measure 400mm × 0.3mm and the males 30mm × 0.2mm). The adults have a lifespan of about 12 years.

Blackfly larvae attach to vegetation or rocks in well oxygenated, flowing water and, since the emerging adults have a limited flight range, heavy infection is associated with areas bordering rivers or streams where blindness rates can exceed 10 per cent of the adult population. In Africa, the most important host species are members of the *S. damnosum* complex. In Central America, the species *S. ochraceum* breeds in small streams in high, coffee-growing areas and bites principally around the head (thus increasing the likelihood of blindness). Figure 2.85 shows the geographical distribution of *Onchocerca*.

Clinical effects

The adult worms become surrounded by fibrous nodules (onchocercomas), usually over bony prominences, but the important pathogenic agents are the microfilariae in the skin.

In the early stages, there is pruritis with an itchy rash and lymphadenopathy in the groin or axilla. After months or years, this can lead to intradermal oedema with pachydermia ('crocodile' skin). Finally, there is loss of elastic fibres causing hernias or 'hanging groin' (hanging lymph glands, Fig. 2.86); atrophy of the skin gives a prematurely aged appearance, with depigmentation resembling leprosy.

'Sowda' is another resulting condition, particularly common in Yemen. It is characterized by hyperpigmentation and thickening of the skin in which there are only a few microfilariae, and by groin lymph node adenopathy.

Blindness is the most important clinical effect and is more common in savanna than in forest areas. It results from two types of lesions in the eyes:

● Anterior lesions, caused by microfilariae reaching the cornea from the skin of the face. When the microfilariae die, they produce a punctate keratitis (fluffy 'snowflake' opacities), sometimes accompanied by chronic conjunctivitis and photophobia. This may be followed by a sclerosing keratitis with an opaque 'apron' spreading from the lower half of the cornea, resulting in complete blindness (Fig. 2.87 upper);

● Posterior lesions in the retina, often with a well-defined patch in both eyes in which all elements have

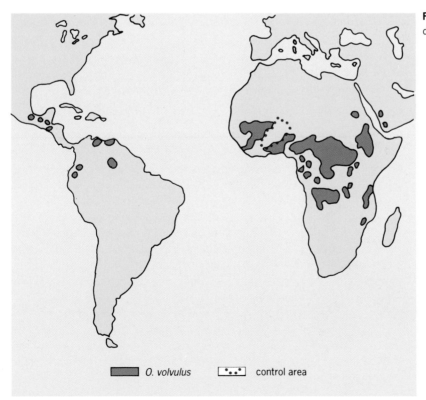

Fig. 2.85 Geographical distribution of *O. volvulus*.

▬▬ *O. volvulus*　　▱•••▱ control area

vanished except the blood vessels (Hissette–Ridley fundus). There is marked sclerosis (hardening) of the choroidal vessels with complete blindness, or just tubular vision remaining (Fig. 2.87 lower). Microfilariae can also cause atrophy of the optic nerve.

Diagnosis

The pruritic rash, typical of the early stages, has to be differentiated from that resulting from other causes, for example scabies, contact dermatitis, insect bites and prickly heat. The presence of nodules, from which portions of worms can be obtained on biopsy, can confirm the diagnosis.

Routine diagnosis is obtained by taking a bloodless snip of skin, measuring about 3mm, using a raised needle and razor blade. This is then gently teased in saline on a microscope slide, left for thirty minutes and examined microscopically (Fig. 2.88) for active microfilariae (these are much more active than those of *M. streptocerca* also found in skin). *O. volvulus* microfilariae measure 250–300μm.

Treatment

DEC kills the microfilariae only and its use has to be repeated weekly to keep their levels low; it also often causes severe itching. Suramin kills adult worms but is no longer recommended due to its toxicity. Ivermectin has been effective at very low doses in clinical trials, and prevents production of microfilariae by the female worms with few side effects. It is now being distributed free in West Africa. Removal of

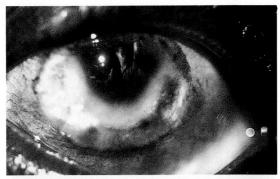

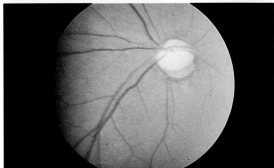

Fig. 2.87 Anterior lesion in the eye caused by *O. volvulus* microfilariae. There is a sclerosing keratitis with an opaque apron spreading from the lower half of the cornea (upper). Posterior lesion in the retina: Hissette–Ridley fundus and marked sclerosis of the choroidal vessels (lower). Courtesy of Dr J Anderson.

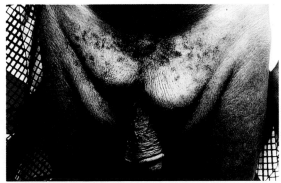

Fig. 2.86 'Hanging groin' and skin changes associated with an *O. volvulus* infection. Courtesy of Prof. G S Nelson.

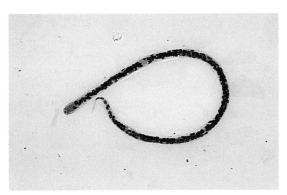

Fig. 2.88 *O. volvulus* microfilaria from a snip of skin. It has no sheath, and is not found in the blood. Note swollen head and lack of nuclei in the tail.

nodules (nodulectomy) is carried out principally in Central America where these are often found on the patient's head.

Prevention and control

Control is principally maintained by destruction of larval *Simulium* with insecticides. A campaign in seven countries of the Volta River basin has interrupted transmission completely in the control area since its inception in 1975, with the use of larvicides sprayed from aeroplanes (see Fig. 3.10) and helicopters, and has now been extended to four others.

The disease was eradicated from Kenya with insecticides effective against *Simulium neavei* larvae which live on the backs of freshwater crabs inhabiting holes in the ground.

Causative organism	Disease
Dracunculus medinensis	Dracunculiasis (guineaworm disease)

Transmission and epidemiology

The mature female worms in the connective tissues provoke a blister on the skin near the anterior end. In a few days, the blister bursts, often after immersion in water, with thousands of larvae being expelled from the rupture of the head-end of the emerging female worm. The larvae measure 600µm and move actively in water. After ingestion by water fleas (*Mesocyclops* and *Thermocyclops* spp., Fig. 2.89), they reach the haemocoele, moult twice, and develop into the infective third stage in about two weeks. When infected cyclops are ingested in drinking water, the released larvae migrate through the intestinal and abdominal walls and reach maturity in the connective tissues in around 3 months.

After fertilization, the males (measuring about 3cm) die, while the females continue to grow (reaching a length of 50–100cm) and become non-feeding

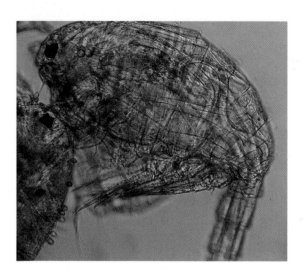

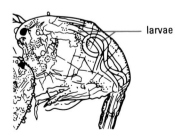

larvae

Fig. 2.89 Cyclops carrying *Dracunculus medinensis* larvae.

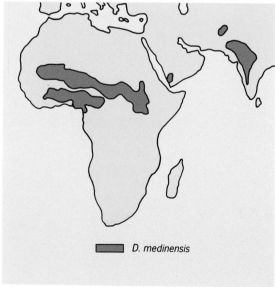

D. medinensis

Fig. 2.90 Geographical distribution of *Dracunculus medinensis*.

'bags', filled with over a million larvae, before they emerge at around one year.

Dracunculus medinensis is found in sub-Saharan Africa and in Asia (Fig. 2.90). Cyclops carrying larvae breed in ponds and open wells, hence dracunculiasis is common in remote rural areas where these are the only sources of drinking water.

Clinical effects

There are usually no symptoms associated with the pre-patent phase until an emerging female worm provokes the formation of a blister, usually on the lower limbs, sometimes preceded by allergic symptoms. In uncomplicated cases, disability lasts only around 4 weeks, until the worm is completely expelled. However, the track of the worm becomes secondarily infected by bacteria in about 50 per cent of cases and disability may last for many months, particularly when large numbers of worms are present (Fig. 2.91). Worms may also burst in the tissues, resulting in a large abscess. Possible sequelae include fibrous ankylosis of joints, contractures of tendons, chronic ulceration, or even tetanus.

Diagnosis

Once the blister forms, there is usually no doubt as to the cause. When it bursts, emerging larvae can be seen under a low-power microscope. IFAT and ELISA tests· may be useful in detecting pre-patent infections but have not been fully evaluated.

Treatment

Various compounds, such as albendazole, mebendazole, niridazole, thiabendazole and metronidazole, appear to act as anti-inflammatory agents, thus allowing worms to be withdrawn more easily.

Prevention and control

Safe drinking supplies should eradicate the disease, as advocated by the 'Clean Drinking Water and Sanitation Decade 1981–1990' campaign. Where this is not possible, control will be maintained by applying measures such as keeping infected individuals away from ponds or step wells to prevent contamination, sieving or boiling drinking water, and the chemical treatment of wells and ponds with Abate (temephos).

Causative organism	Disease
Trichinella spiralis	Trichiniasis

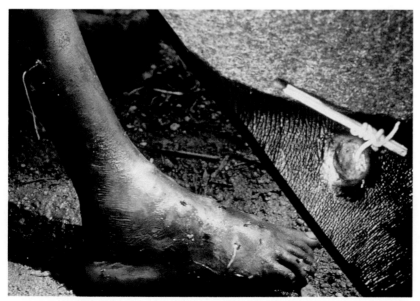

Fig. 2.91 Dracunculiasis. Female worms emerging from the leg and foot of a girl with secondary bacterial invasion (cellulitis), causing severe disability (left). An emerging female worm being wound out on a matchstick, about five centimetres a day (right).

Transmission and epidemiology

This is a zoonotic infection and the life cycle can be maintained in a wide range of animals (Fig. 2.92). In most parts of the world, human infection is contracted from the domestic pig (hog). The adults are minute worms living partially embedded in the mucosa of the ileum. The females measure 2.8mm in length, and the males 1.1mm. Each female produces up to two thousand larvae during its lifespan which is less than 8 weeks.

The first-stage larvae penetrate the intestinal wall and are carried into the muscle cells where they coil up and become infective to a new host within 3 weeks. If the larvae are ingested by a new host in undercooked meat, they are released, enter the intestinal mucosa, moult 4 times and develop into adults in around 30 hours. Thus, there are no free-living stages and the same animal (or person) acts both as final and intermediate host.

Trichinella infections in animals occur worldwide, but infections in man are more widespread in Eastern Europe (4 percent prevalence in Poland), the Arctic region inhabited by Eskimo people (up to 50 percent prevalence), Asia, South America and East Africa.

Clinical effects

The adult worms cause small haemorrhages and can give rise to diarrhoea and abdominal pains. In light infections, larvae cause muscle pains and eosinophilia but in heavy infections symptoms mimic influenza or typhoid, with periorbital and generalized muscular oedema (Fig. 2.93). There may also be pulmonary, nervous system and cardiac involvement. Severe muscular pain may last for months, if death does not intervene.

Diagnosis

The clinical signs and symptoms tend to be more definite where there is epidemic infection. Within 4 weeks after infection, encysted larvae can be found in muscle biopsies. Immunological tests include CF, IFAT and ELISA. Commercial kits for bentonite

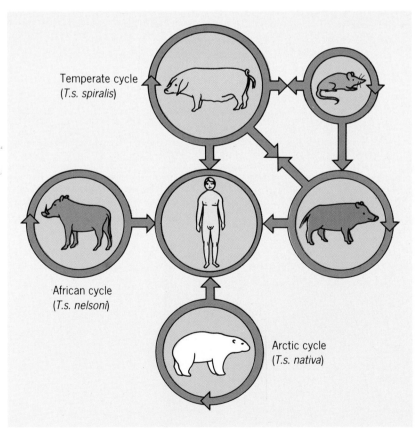

Fig. 2.92 There are different types of life cycle of *Trichinella spiralis* in animals in various parts of the world; thus, the parasites are often regarded as different subspecies, as shown.

Temperate cycle
(*T.s. spiralis*)

African cycle
(*T.s. nelsoni*)

Arctic cycle
(*T.s. nativa*)

flocculation, latex agglutination and intradermal tests are available.

Treatment
Mebendazole is the best treatment against muscle larvae (thiabendazole is no longer recommended, because of related allergic reactions). When neurological symptoms occur, massive doses of corticosteroids are given for several weeks. Adult worms can be treated with levamisole or pyrantel pamoate.

Prevention and control
Larvae in pigs can be destroyed by heat (above 60°C)

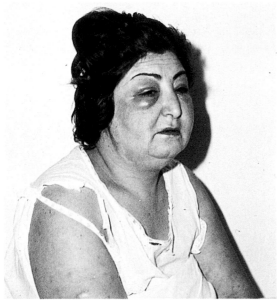

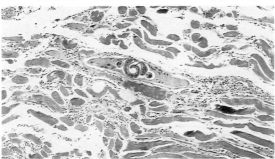

Fig. 2.93 Periorbital and generalized oedema in a *Trichinella spiralis* infection, courtesy of Dr Kemal Arab (above). Section of skeletal muscle from a fatal case of trichiniasis, showing swelling and oedema of the muscle fibres with acute inflammation (myositis) caused by larvae. A few weeks after infection, the larvae become encapsulated in a cyst (below).

or by deep freezing. At the abattoir, acid pepsin digested muscle samples from many pigs can be routinely examined under the microscope for larvae.

Laws preventing the feeding of uncooked waste food (swill) to pigs have almost eradicated the disease in the United States (from 16 percent infection in 1950, to only 109 reported clinical cases by 1970).

Causative organism	Disease
Angiostrongylus cantonensis	Eosinophilic meningitis
Gnathostoma spinigerum	High eosinophilia, oedema

Transmission and epidemiology
Angiostrongylus cantonensis is found in the Pacific Islands, Southeast Asia and Cuba. The infection in man is zoonotic; adults (related to hookworms) are normally found in the lungs of rats. Larvae hatch out from eggs passed by rats and develop in snails and slugs. When these are eaten, either on purpose (the giant African snail is a popular delicacy) or by mistake, the larvae penetrate the intestinal wall and reach the brain via the blood, but do not develop further. In the brain, they cause inflammatory lesions resulting in vomiting, headache, neck stiffness and sometimes paralysis (Fig. 2.94). There is high eosinophilia in the cerebrospinal fluid.

A similar parasite exists in Central and South America (*A. costaricensis*) which does not attack the brain but causes lesions in the intestinal wall.

Gnathostoma spinigerum is found in many Asian countries. The infection in man is zoonotic and the

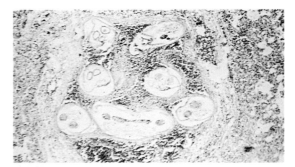

Fig. 2.94 Larvae of *Angiostrongylus cantonensis* in microscopic section of human brain, surrounded by an intense granulomatous reaction.

natural hosts are fish-eating carnivores. The larvae which hatch out from eggs are passed in the faeces of cats or dogs, develop in cyclops and finally in fish. When fish are eaten raw, the larvae penetrate the intestinal wall and reach the subcutis where they can cause a migrating oedema similar to loiasis (Fig. 2.95). Occasionally, they attack the eyes or brain with an accompanying high eosinophilia.

Larvae do not mature in man.

LARVA MIGRANS

This term is used to describe larvae which do not mature in humans but wander in the human body, sometimes with serious results.

Possible causes of visceral larva migrans (VLM), such as *Gnathostoma* (and occasionally other members of the same group, the spirurids), *Angiostrongylus*, *Anisakis*, fly larvae and *Spirometra*, are considered in the appropriate sections.

Causative organism	Disease
Toxocara canis (dog roundworm)	Visceral larva migrans (VLM)

Eggs, passed in the faeces of young dogs, are widely distributed in the soil of most parts of the world, and when ingested by children, the hatched second-stage larvae penetrate the gut wall and undergo a similar migration to those of *Ascaris*. *Toxocara* larvae do not mature in man, however, and being thinner, can sometimes pass through the sinusoids and disperse to the kidneys, brain or eyes. It is not known if two other common ascarids of pets, *T. cati* and *Toxascaris leonina*, are involved.

The larvae usually end up in the liver where they elicit a strong inflammatory response, and each becomes surrounded by an eosinophilic microabscess which eventually fibroses to give a granuloma. Overt disease is very rare and consists of long-lasting hepatomegaly, hypereosinophilia (up to 60 per cent) and raised gammaglobulins with brief pulmonary and generalized allergic manifestations. Larvae in the brain have resulted in epilepsy, and in the eye to retinal lesions (Fig. 2.96), which have been mistaken for retinoblastoma and the eye removed.

Diagnosis is by ELISA or IFAT; treatment by DEC or thiabendazole. Although a high proportion of children in many countries show the presence of *Toxocara* antibodies, clinical symptoms are rare.

Causative organism	Disease
Ancylostoma braziliensis, *A. caninum* and *A. ceylanicum* (dog hookworms)	Cutaneous larva migrans; creeping eruption

When the infective filariform larvae of some animal hookworms penetrate the skin of man from contaminated ground, they follow a tortuous path under the skin, causing an erythrematous, inflammatory reaction with intense itching which can last for weeks. Treatment is with an ethyl chloride spray or with thiabendazole. A similar effect can occur following the penetration of the cercariae of bird schistosomes in water.

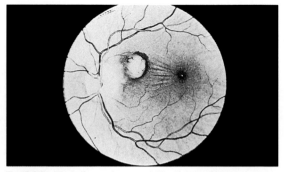

Fig. 2.95 Oedematous reaction above eye caused by migrating third-stage larva of *Gnathostoma spinigerum*. The oedema usually lasts about two weeks. Courtesy of Dr P Jayaneta.

Fig. 2.96 View of eye of young child with granuloma surrounding a larva of *Toxocara canis*. Courtesy of Prof. N A Ashton.

3. ARTHROPODS

group	genus	disease
Order Diptera		
Family Culicidae Mosquitoes	*Anopheles*	Malaria Lymphatic filariasis (*Wuchereria*)
	Culex	Lymphatic filariasis
	Aedes	Lymphatic filariasis Yellow fever
	Mansonia	Lymphatic filariasis (*Brugia*)
Family Psychodidae Sandflies	*Phlebotomus* *Lutzomyia* *Psychodopygus*	Leishmaniasis
Family Simuliidae Simuliids	*Simulium*	Onchocerciasis (Ozzardi filariasis)
Family Ceratopogonidae Ceratopogonids	*Culicoides*	Ozzardi filariasis Perstans filariasis Streptocerciasis
Family Glossinidae Tsetse flies	*Glossina*	Sleeping sickness
Family Tabanidae Tabanid flies	*Chrysops*	Loiasis
Order Siphonaptera		
Family Pulicidae Lice	*Pediculus*	Epidemic typhus Trench fever Epidemic relapsing fever
Order Anoplura		
Family Pediculidae Fleas	*Xenopsylla*	Plague Endemic typhus Dwarf tapeworm
	Ctenocephalides	Dog tapeworm
Order Hemiptera		
Family Reduviidae Triatomine bugs	*Triatoma* *Rhodnius* *Panstrongylus*	Chagas' disease

Fig. 3.1 Parasitic diseases transmitted by insects.

The phylum Arthropoda contains more than 85 per cent of all known animals. Members are characterized by having a segmented body covered by a protective exoskeleton.

The class Insecta includes many forms which are blood feeders on man and can thus transmit many important parasitic and other infectious diseases (Fig. 3.1). Insects are characterized by having the body divided into a head, a thorax and an abdomen and have three pairs of legs. There are typically two (or in the order Diptera, only one) pairs of wings, although the fleas and lice have no wings. The head has a pair of antennae and one or two pairs of palps.

The class Arachnida have no antennae or wings and four pairs of legs. Ticks and mites are the most important groups which have members feeding on the blood of man.

The class Crustacea have two pairs of antennae and at least five pairs of legs. They are mostly aquatic and members act as intermediate hosts, for example, crabs and crayfish are host to *Paragonimus*, while copepods are host to *Diphyllobothrium* and *Dracunculus*.

MOSQUITOES

The two subfamilies of mosquito can be distinguished as shown in Fig. 3.2. Only female mosquitoes feed on blood and therefore only they can act as vectors of parasites. Only anophelines

transmit human malaria, but other species of *Plasmodium* (those infecting birds and rodents) may be transmitted by culicines also.

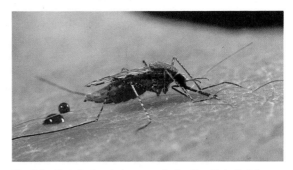

Fig. 3.3 Female *Anopheles* mosquito feeding. Note that the body is usually held at an angle of about 45° to the surface of the skin and the maxillary palps are long. Male mosquitoes, which do not feed on blood, can be differentiated from females because the antennae are feathery. Courtesy of Mr C J Webb.

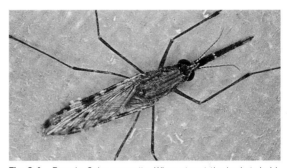

Fig. 3.4 Female *Culex* mosquito. When at rest the body is held parallel to the surface. The palps are much shorter than the proboscis, although they cannot be clearly seen in this specimen.

	Anophelinae	**Culicinae**
Egg:	air floats on each side	no lateral air floats
Larvae:	rest parallel to water surface; breathing tube (siphon) absent	rest at an angle to water surface; breathing tube (siphon) present
Adults:	abdomen not banded. Rest with body at an acute angle to surface	abdomen usually with transverse light and dark bands. Rest with body parallel to surface

Fig. 3.2 Characteristics used to distinguish between mosquitoes of the subfamilies Anophelinae and Culicinae.

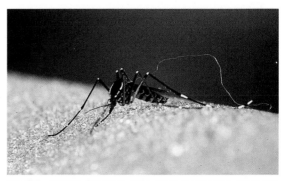

Fig. 3.5 Female *Aedes* mosquito. Most species have black and white rings on the legs and patterns on the thorax. Otherwise similar to *Culex* except for differences in the wing veins. Courtesy of Professor W W MacDonald.

Life cycle

Female *Anopheles*, *Culex* and *Aedes* are shown in Figs 3.3–3.5. Fertilized females lay their eggs in stagnant water in pools, ponds, buckets, empty cans and other objects which may hold water. *Anopheles* and *Aedes* eggs are laid singly, though those of *Anopheles* may be grouped in rosettes; *Culex* eggs are glued together to form 'rafts'. The speed of development depends on the species and the ambient temperature, but usually eggs hatch after a few days to release an actively swimming and feeding larva. The larva (Fig. 3.6) breathes air through posterior spiracles (which in Culicinae are placed at the tip of a breathing tube or siphon), and so when at rest lies near the water surface. After a week or two, the larvae moult to become pupae. The pupae do not feed but move actively; they also breathe air, through a pair of small dorsal tubes called respiratory trumpets, and so rest near the water surface. After a further few days, the adults emerge from the pupae. *Mansonia* is unusual as both larvae and pupae obtain oxygen by inserting their siphons or respiratory trumpets into the stems of water plants.

Species

Many species of the genera listed in Fig. 3.1 can transmit the respective parasites.

Many species of several genera, in both subfamilies, can transmit *Wuchereria bancrofti* (see p.105). *Mansonia* is the main vector of *Brugia malayi* (p.105), but species of *Anopheles* and *Aedes* can also transmit this nematode in some areas. *Aedes* (and some other genera) are notorious as the vectors of yellow fever and dengue viruses.

Control

Control can be directed at larvae and pupae, by draining breeding sites, or by spreading a film of oil on the water surface, which prevents the larvae and pupae (except for those of *Mansonia*) from breathing, or by adding insecticides to the water; species of fish which feed on mosquito larvae have sometimes been used to control mosquitoes.

Adult mosquitoes can be attacked by residual insecticide sprays, though they are becoming alarmingly resistant to many of these. Individual persons can protect themselves by screening windows, using the traditional bed nets, and using 'knock-down' sprays and coils in houses.

SANDFLIES

Sandflies are very small Diptera (2–5mm long) of the family Psychodidae, subfamily Phlebotominae, with hairy wings. When not flying, the wings are held almost vertically (like a V) above the back, not folded (like the blades of a pair of scissors) as in many other insects (Fig. 3.7). (In the Caribbean region, the term 'sandfly' is applied to midges of the genus *Culicoides*.)

Only female sandflies feed on blood, so only they can act as vectors; males and females also feed on sugary plant secretions.

Life cycle

Fertilized females lay up to 70 or so minute eggs singly in damp soil, decaying organic matter, animal burrows, or similar places (not in water), and the

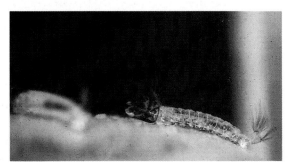

Fig. 3.6 *Anopheles* larva.

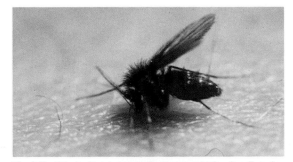

Fig. 3.7 Minute American sandfly (*Lutzomyia*) feeding. Females feed on blood every 3–4 days at night. They are weak fliers with a characteristic hopping type of flight. They cannot bite through clothes. Courtesy of Dr R P Lane.

eggs hatch after a few days. The small, white caterpillar-like larvae feed on decaying organic material; they undergo three moults, the last (some 4–6 weeks after hatching in tropical species) giving rise to pupae. After a further 1 to 2 weeks, the adult emerges from the pupa. Adult females probably survive for 2 or 3 weeks under natural conditions.

Species

Five genera and around 400 species are known, but the vectors of human leishmaniasis (p.37) all belong to the genera *Phlebotomus* (in Europe, Africa and Asia), and to *Lutzomyia* (in Central and South America).

Control

Spraying inside houses with residual insecticides protects against only the few species of sandflies which, as yet, have not developed significant resistance.

Netting screens over windows and bed nets can be used, but must be very fine to prevent their entry. Ordinary mosquito nets are inadequate, though if they are impregnated with repellant they may be effective. Sandfly bites can be prevented to some extent by wearing long trousers and long-sleeved shirts during dusk and at night (especially out of doors), when sandflies usually feed. Repellants can be applied to exposed skin.

SIMULIUM

Common names: blackflies, buffalo gnats,
coffee flies.

Blackflies have a worldwide distribution and *Simulium* is the principal genus in the family Simuliidae, responsible for transmitting the filarial nematode *Onchocerca volvulus* (p.111).

The adults are small (1.5–4mm) and stout with a humped thorax. African vectors are black in colour but South American vectors are orange (Fig. 3.8). The head has a pair of large compound eyes, separated on top of the head in females. The antennae are short and stout, and the mouthparts are also short so they do not penetrate very deeply into the skin; only the female flies bite. By a scissor-like rasping action they cut through the skin, rupture minor capillaries and produce a small pool of blood. In this way, microfilariae of *O. volvulus* in the skin are able to enter the fly.

Life cycle

Eggs are laid in running water but the type of breeding place varies from fast flowing large rivers (as in the Volta, Niger, Nile and Congo and their branches in Africa) to small trickles of water depending on the species. Eggs are usually laid on rocks, stones or vegetation, a few hundred at a time, in a sticky mass or string just below the surface. Eggs hatch in about one day and there are 6–8 larval instars.

Larvae remain attached under the water and are filter-feeders, with the aid of large mouth brushes, on suspended food particles (Fig. 3.9). After one or two weeks, a cocoon is woven and an attached pupa with two large, branched breathing tubes formed. Several days later, the young adult emerges in an air bubble.

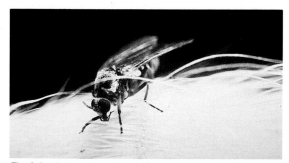

Fig. 3.8 A female *Simulium*. These are small but stout insects with a marked hump on the thorax and no scales on the wings. They are pool feeders with scarifying mouthparts.

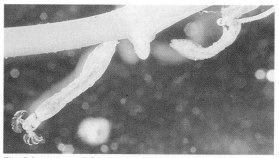

Fig. 3.9 Larvae of *Simulium* on vegetation in fast flowing water. These attached larvae are filter feeders with the aid of the large mouth brushes visible at the unattached end. Courtesy of Dr A E Bianco.

Species

The most important vector species for human onchocerciasis in Africa is *Simulium damnosum*. Recent studies indicate that this is a species complex with at least 40 cytologically different forms, some of which live in savanna areas and some in forest. While most have a flight range of only a few kilometres from their breeding sites, the important savanna forms can travel long distances.

The larvae of *S. neavei* attach to freshwater crabs and onchocerciasis was eradicated from Kenya by the use of DDT against the larvae, particularly in the holes occupied by crabs.

In Central America, the principal vector is *S. ochraceum* which breeds in very small streams, particularly in well-wooded coffee fincas between 1000 and 2000m above sea level. It is a very efficient vector but has a short flight range and has a preference for biting the upper half of the body, which may account for the localization of onchocercal nodules on the head in Mexico and Guatemala, with increased risk of blindness. *S. metallicum* is a zoophilic species, principally biting the legs, which breeds in streams and rivers. It is a major vector only in Venezuela where eye lesions are uncommon. In Brazil, *S. amazonicum* transmits *Mansonella ozzardi* (but see p.123).

Control

A very large onchocerciasis control programme involving many countries in the Volta river basin in West Africa started in 1974 and has been based almost entirely on the aerial application of larval insecticides (principally temephos) (Fig. 3.10). Almost complete control of flies has been obtained in Burkina Faso, Niger, eastern Mali and northern savanna regions of Ivory Coast, Ghana, Togo and Benin, and the programme is being extended westwards and southwards. No children have been infected with onchocerciasis in the centre of the control area in the last few years, severe eye lesions have fallen dramatically and adult worms in infected people are now dying.

CULICOIDES

Common names: biting midges, punkies,
no-see-ums, gnats, 'sandflies'
(Caribbean).

Culicoides, belonging to the family Ceratopogonidae, are found in both tropical and subarctic areas and can transmit the human filarial parasites *Mansonella perstans*, *M. streptocerca* and *M. ozzardi*.

Adults are very small (1.5–5mm) and only the females bite man (Fig. 3.11). The mouthparts are similar to those of simuliids, so they are also pool feeders.

Life cycle

Eggs are laid in batches on rotting vegetation, soil,

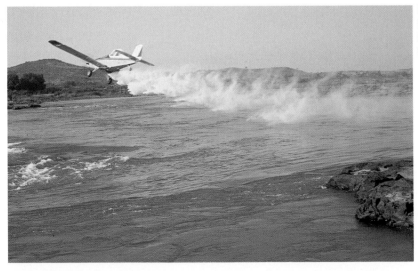

Fig. 3.10 Control of *Simulium* larvae with aerial application of insecticide (temephos) to a river in West Africa. Courtesy of WHO.

mud or the edges of salt-water marshes, depending on species. Eggs usually hatch within a few days and there are four larval instars. Larvae feed on decaying vegetable matter and convert to pupae in 2–4 weeks in the tropics. Adults hatch out from the cocoon in about one week.

Adults have a short flight range of a few hundred metres from their breeding sites and often swarms bite exposed parts of the body, particularly in the evening, causing severe irritation.

Species

Culicoides milnei and *C. grahami* transmit *M. perstans*, and the latter species *M. streptocerca* also in Africa. Both midges breed in rotting banana stumps. *C. furens* is the principal vector of *M. ozzardi*.

Control

Control of biting midges is not easy although sometimes habitats can be drained or flooded. Larval insecticides have been used successfully in some areas.

TSETSE FLIES

Tsetse flies are large Diptera (6–14mm long) of the family Glossinidae, which are restricted to tropical Africa. They are dull brownish-grey in colour (Fig. 3.12). Both sexes feed exclusively on blood, so both have their mouthparts modified to form a piercing and sucking proboscis. They can be distinguished from other, rather similar flies (such as horse flies) by the so-called 'hatchet cell' formed by some of the wing veins.

Life cycle

Tsetse flies are unusual as they do not lay eggs but deposit, one at a time, mature larvae which burrow into soil or other material. Almost immediately the larval cuticle becomes hardened and dark brown or black in colour to form a protective shell or puparium. After around 4 days, the larva pupates, still within the puparium.

Female tsetse mate only once, within a few days of emerging from the puparium; live sperm are stored for the rest of the female's life. The first larva is deposited usually about 2–3 weeks later; thereafter they follow at fairly regular intervals of about 10–14 days, the timing depending on the species of fly and the ambient temperature.

The length of time before an adult emerges from the pupa also depends on the temperature; it usually ranges from about 3 to 4½ weeks. Under ideal conditions, adult female tsetse may live for up to 6 months; under natural conditions longevity is considerably reduced, perhaps to 7–10 days. Males and females have a meal of blood every 2–3 days; they will feed on a fairly wide range of mammals (including man), but different species have their more favoured hosts.

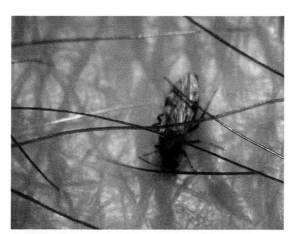

Fig. 3.11 Minute feeding female *Culicoides*. At rest the typically patterned wings are placed over the abdomen like closed scissor blades.

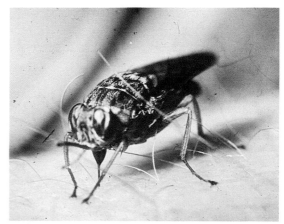

Fig. 3.12 Tsetse fly, *Glossina morsitans* feeding. Courtesy of Dr W Petana.

Species

Twenty-two species of *Glossina* are known; they fall into three groups, named after their best known species as the *G. fusca*, *G. palpalis* and *G. morsitans* groups. Probably all species can act as vectors of trypanosomiasis (p.27), but the more important vectors are shown in Fig. 3.13. Flies of the *G. morsitans* group can tolerate drier conditions than can the *G. palpalis* group, and are therefore more widely distributed over the vast areas of East African savanna; the *G. palpalis* group are more restricted to moist forest and, especially, river banks and lake shores in East and West Africa.

Control

Early attempts to control tsetse were based on eradication of their favoured mammalian blood-meal sources, but such methods are expensive and ecologically undesirable. Other methods which have been, and to some extent still are, used include destruction of the habitat by selective bush clearing and tree felling, and spraying with insecticides. The latter is most effective when used against species such as *G. palpalis*, which has a limited habitat range; river bank vegetation can be sprayed reasonably economically from a small boat. Aerial spraying against wider-ranging species, such as *G. morsitans*, can be done, but is very expensive and so can be used in rather limited areas only.

A recent development has been the use of traps which are impregnated with chemicals found in the breath of oxen, which are very attractive to tsetse flies and so enormously increase the efficiency of the traps.

The best means of tsetse control, where it is economically and sociologically feasible, is to encourage agricultural land-use; farming and other human activities are incompatible with the continued existence of tsetse flies. Problems arise, however, where it has been decided to preserve large areas of Africa in their 'natural condition', as wild animal reserves and parks.

Further details of all these methods (and others) can be found in the books listed as further reading.

CHRYSOPS

Common names: softly-softly fly, mango fly.

Chrysops belongs to the family Tabanidae (subfamily Chrysopsinae) which includes the ubiquitous horse-flies and deerflies. It is approximately the same size as a tsetse fly but, at rest, the wings are separated like an open pair of scissors, as in house flies (Fig. 3.14).

Males feed exclusively on sugars from plants while females feed on blood from a wide variety of animals. Females bite mainly during the day and are powerful

Group	Glossina palpalis	G. morsitans	G. fusca
Important vectors	G. palpalis G. tachinoides G. fuscipes	G. morsitans G. pallidipes	flies rarely feed on man
Parasite transmitted	Trypanosoma brucei gambiense	T. brucei including 'rhodesiense' forms	

Fig. 3.13 Species of *Glossina* important in transmitting trypanosomiasis.

flyers. The mouthparts of the female flies are highly adapted for rasping and piercing skin, and unlike those of tsetse flies always point downwards from the head. The blood is lapped up from the painful puncture wound.

Life cycle

Around 100–500 eggs are deposited on the underside of leaves, twigs or rocks overhanging muddy forest streams. Larvae hatch in around one week and drop into the water. Larvae scavenge on detritus and take up to a year before they pupate, with probably seven moults.

The pupa is partially buried in mud and the adult emerges in 1–3 weeks.

Species

C. silacea and *C. dimidiata* are the most important vectors of loiasis (p.110) in West Africa and *C. distinctipennis* in Central Africa.

Other tabanids are important pest nuisances and can mechanically transmit tularaemia and some animal trypanosomes.

Control

Larval insecticiding is not usually successful because of the difficulties in locating breeding places. Personal protection is afforded by insect repellants.

MYIASIS

Myiasis is the invasion of human and other vertebrate tissues by fly larvae of the order Diptera. Larvae may attack cutaneous tissues, body cavities such as the eyes and nose, or the gut and urogenital system.

Myiasis may be obligatory, when it is essential for the larvae to live on a host for a part of their life (a group including species of the genera *Wohlfahrtia*, *Cochliomyia*, *Auchmeromyia*, *Chrysomya*, *Cordylobia*, *Dermatobia*, *Hypoderma*, *Oestrus* and *Gasterophilus*), or facultative, when the larvae are usually free-living or feed on carcasses but can sometimes attack living hosts (a group including species of *Sarcophaga*, *Calliphora*, *Lucilia* and *Phormia*).

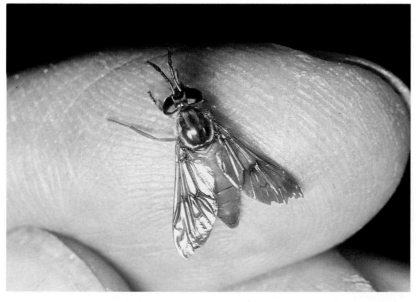

Fig. 3.14 The large, sturdy, tabanid biting fly, *Chrysops*. The wings have bands of colour and characteristic patterns of veins.

The identification of fly larvae in the body can be difficult; the structure of the spiracles (breathing organs) at the tail end is a very important feature in diagnosis as is the presence and arrangement of bristles (these can make extraction difficult). Removed larvae should be killed in hot water and preserved in 80 per cent alcohol for identification by an expert. The common names, distribution and usual hosts of the flies which have larvae attacking man are shown in Fig. 3.15 and the most important are discussed below.

Dermatobia hominis

Dermatobia hominis adults are metallic blue flies which occur principally on the edges of tropical forests over most of Central and South America. The females catch mosquitoes and biting flies and glue eggs to them. When these attack a mammal to obtain a blood

name of fly	family	distribution	popular name	site of larvae in body	reservoir hosts
Dermatobia hominis	Cuterebridae	Central & South America	Neotropical bot or warble fly	Subcutaneous	Cattle & other mammals
Cochliomyia hominivorax	Calliphoridae	North & South America	New World screw worm	Subcutaneous from wounds and sores	Cattle, sheep, horses, goats
Chrysomya bezziana	Calliphoridae	Asia & Africa	Old World screw worm	Subcutaneous, usually from wounds & sores	Cattle, sheep, horses, goats
Cordylobia anthropophaga	Calliphoridae	Africa	Tumbu fly	Subcutaneous	Dogs, rodents, monkeys
Auchmeromyia luteola	Calliphoridae	Africa	Congo floor maggot	Blood feeding (not true myiasis)	Warthogs
Lucilia species	Calliphoridae	Worldwide	Greenbottles	Wounds	Usually on meat or carcasses
Calliphora species	Calliphoridae	Worldwide	Bluebottles	Wounds	Usually on meat or carcasses
Phormia species	Calliphoridae	Temperate regions	Blowflies	Wounds	Usually on meat or carcasses
Oestrus ovis	Oestridae	Worldwide	Gad fly	Nasal cavity & eyes	Sheep
Hypoderma bovis	Oestridae	Northern hemisphere	Cattle warble	Subcutaneous with migration	Cattle
Wohlfahrtia magnifica	Sarcophagidae	Southern Europe Asia, North Africa	Old World flesh fly	Body cavities & sores	Domestic & farm animals
W. vigil	Sarcophagidae	North America	New World flesh fly	Subcutaneous (children)	Pets & wild animals
Sarcophaga species	Sarcophagidae	Worldwide	Flesh flies	Wounds	Usually on meat or carcasses
Gasterophilus intestinalis	Gasterophilidae	Worldwide	Bot fly	Subcutaneous	Horses

Fig. 3.15 Flies causing myiasis in man.

meal, one or more larvae emerge from the eggs and penetrate the skin. Larvae grow in separate subcutaneous pockets with a breathing pore to the outside and the posterior end of a larva can be seen in each, with two small brown spiracles (Fig. 3.16). Larvae moult twice and after 6–12 weeks the third-stage instars wriggle out of the skin and pupate under the soil.

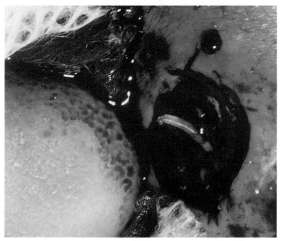

Fig. 3.16 Extraction of a single larva of *Dermatobia hominis*. The posterior portion of the larva, which acts as a breathing tube, is visible before extraction. The stouter anterior portion is covered with spines and is very difficult to remove. Courtesy of Dr R P Lane.

Larvae produce boil-like swellings which continually ooze pus and can be very painful. Occasionally ocular, or sometimes fatal cerebral, myiasis can occur. Larvae are best removed with forceps after opening up the lesion surgically. The usual hosts are cattle and human infections are most common in cattle workers and in children.

Cochliomyia hominivorax

Cochliomyia hominivorax is widely distributed in the Americas. The metallic green female flies glue eggs in masses to clean skin near to a wound or scratch, or occasionally on mucous membranes of the nose, mouth or vagina.

The hatched larval maggots tunnel deeply and produce a communal boil-like lesion which is extremely painful and becomes secondarily infected, leading to severe mutilation or even death in around 8 per cent of cases (Fig. 3.17). After around one week of feeding, the mature maggots exit and drop to the ground to pupate.

This fly is an important parasite of cattle but has been eliminated from most of the United States by the massive release of sterile irradiated males.

Chrysomya bezziana

Chrysomya bezziana is a large metallic blue fly with a green thorax found in Asia where most human cases of *Chrysomya* myiasis occur and in Africa south of the Sahara (Fig. 3.18). Females lay numerous eggs in the nasal cavities and other mucous membranes or

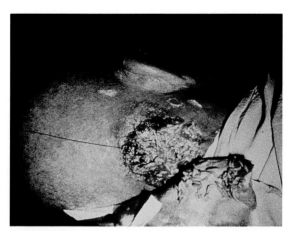

Fig. 3.17 Over 400 larvae of the New World screw-worm *Cochliomyia hominivorax* in a fatal lesion in the hind brain of a man in Central America. Courtesy of Dr R B Holliman.

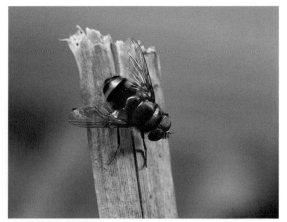

Fig. 3.18 Adult Old World screw worm fly *Chrysomya*. The body is a metallic green colour.

in wounds and cause deep, foul-smelling necrotic lesions which can cause considerable disfigurement if the face is attacked. They can be treated by adding 15 per cent chloroform in vegetable oil and the emergent larvae removed with forceps.

Cordylobia anthropophaga (tumbu fly)

Cordylobia anthropophaga is a large yellow-brown fly found throughout Africa south of the Sahara. The female lays eggs on sandy ground contaminated with urine or often on washed and drying clothes. The larvae penetrate unbroken skin and cause the formation of solitary, boil-like swellings from which they emerge in around 12 days and pupate on the ground. Larvae maintain a breathing aperture to the surface and can be induced to emerge by covering with petroleum jelly.

Wohlfahrtia

Wohlfahrtia magnifica are greyish, hairy flies occurring in southern Europe, North Africa and Asia, which can deposit numerous larvae (not eggs) in the ear, nose and eyes of man or on broken skin. The larvae live in open wounds and sometimes burrow deeply causing great disfigurement. *W. vigil* occurs in North America as far south as Ohio and is attracted to purulent discharges or soiled nappies (diapers) of young children. Lesions tend to be more superficial than those of *W. magnifica*. Larvae of *Sarcophaga* species usually feed only on necrotic tissue if they attack wounds but are occasionally swallowed and cause abdominal pain before they are passed out.

Oestrus ovis

Oestrus ovis, the sheep nasal bot or gad fly, has a worldwide distribution and can cause ophthalmic myiasis, particularly in North Africa and eastern USSR. The female flies drop their eggs into the orbit and cause painful inflammation, although fortunately larvae do not develop fully in man.

Other flies causing myiasis in man

Larvae of many flies normally associated with carrion, such as *Lucilia*, *Calliphora*, *Phormia*, or even house-flies (*Musca* and *Fannia*) sometimes attack necrotic tissue in wounds, and very occasionally surrounding healthly tissue also.

As with *Oestrus ovis*, the larvae of other flies attacking domestic animals, such as *Hypoderma* or *Gasterophilus*, may invade the orbit.

FLEAS

There are many thousand species of fleas, belonging to the order Siphonaptera, but only a few are important pests and vectors to man.

Adult fleas are small (2–3mm), oval insects, compressed laterally and with long legs for hopping and jumping. Both sexes have a proboscis adapted for piercing skin and sucking blood, and take frequent blood meals (Fig. 3.19).

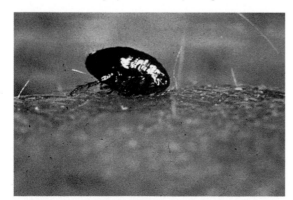

Fig. 3.19 The rat flea *Xenopsylla* feeding (both sexes feed on blood). Fleas are compressed laterally and the mid pair of legs are specialized for jumping. There are no wings but the body and legs are covered in small spines.

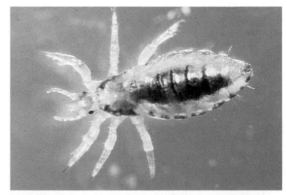

Fig. 3.20 Fed adult louse *Pediculus*. Both sexes suck blood and are flattened dorso-ventrally and have no wings. Courtesy of Dr R Robinson.

Life cycle

The impregnated female deposits the sticky eggs on the ground or in infested nests. There are 3 larval instars which feed principally on organic debris, including dried blood and adult faeces, before a cocoon is formed. The adult in the cocoon can survive for up to a year. Although there are human, cat, dog and rat fleas, they are not very specific and all may bite man if the normal hosts are absent.

Species

Fleas associated with man include:

- *Pulex irritans*, the human flea.

- *Xenopsylla cheopis*, the ubiquitous rat flea. This species is responsible for the transmission of bubonic plague (*Yersinia pestis*) and endemic or murine typhus (*Rickettsia mooseri*). It could also transmit the tapeworm *Hymenolepis diminuta*, occasionally found in children (see p.83).

- *Ctenocephalides canis* and *C. felis* infest dogs and cats in temperate countries and transmit the tapeworm *Dipylidium caninum.*

- *Tunga penetrans*, the jigger or chigoe, is a parasite of man and other animals in tropical America and Africa. Eggs are dropped by females on the floor of houses or on the ground outside, and larvae reach adulthood in around 18 days. Both sexes, measuring around 1mm, bite the skin of the feet but the female, after fertilization, burrows into the skin where it is soft, e.g. between the toes or under the toenail, leaving a small hole for breathing, defaecating and passing out numerous eggs. The abdomen becomes enormously enlarged inside the tissues to the size of a pea (6mm). The area around the flea becomes itchy and inflamed, and secondary infection is common. Females should be teased out with a sterilized needle as soon as possible before they swell.

Control

The control of domestic fleas is often difficult and involves frequent use of pyrethroids around the whole house and must be carefully coordinated with the control of rats in the case of *Xenopsylla*.

LICE

The three types of sucking lice which attack man are members of the order Anoplura. Lice spend their whole life cycle on or near the host, both sexes feeding on blood, and leave it only to transfer to another similar host. They have very strict host specificity.

Species

- *Pediculus humanus capitis*, the head louse, is found only on the hair of the head of man and measures 2–4mm in length. It has curved teeth around the mouth for holding the skin and 3 small stylets for piercing it (Fig. 3.20).

In the developed world, 2–10 per cent of school children have head lice but these days infestations are usually light, with only moderate itching of the scalp caused by sensitization to louse saliva. When large numbers of lice are present, however, there may be fever and aches, and often secondary infection of the lesions, including impetigo, which can be carried by the louse.

Diagnosis is usually by finding live lice or empty egg shells (known as nits and measuring 0.8×0.3mm) attached to hairs, often behind the ears.

- *Pediculus humanus humanus*, the body louse, is almost identical to the head louse but lives in clothing and visits the skin only to feed. The body louse can transmit various diseases. The highly pathogenic louse-borne epidemic typhus is caused by *Rickettsia prowazeki* which multiples in the cells of the louse gut. Man becomes infected when louse faeces are rubbed into the abrasion or membranes of eye and mouth. It kills the louse in about 12 days. Trench fever is an incapacitating disease which was particularly prevalent in soldiers in the two world wars. It is caused by *R. quintana* which multiplies in the louse gut and infection is from a crushed louse or from its faeces; probably also from inhalation of dried louse faeces in dust.

Louse-borne epidemic relapsing fever is caused by *Borrelia recurrentis.* When a louse bites an infected individual, the spirochaetes ingested with the blood meal penetrate into the haemocoele and multiply. Another person can be infected only when a crushed louse is rubbed into an abrasion or perhaps when one is cracked between the teeth.

● *Pthirus pubis*, crab lice, are small (up to 2mm) lice preferring widely-spaced coarse hairs; they are often found on pubic hair or, in children, on eyelashes or eyebrows. The adult may remain at the base of a single hair and is very difficult to see.

Transmission is usually by sexual contact.

Control

The eggs of body lice are usually laid on underclothes and this louse can be easily eliminated by thorough washing of clothing in hot water above 60°C, so infestation is common only under conditions of poor hygiene.

Treatment of all lice is with malathion, carbaryl or pyrethroid lotions.

TRIATOMINE BUGS

Common names: kissing bugs, assassin bugs, cone-nosed bugs

Kissing bugs (so named because they often bite around the lips of their victims) are large insects with four wings (order Hemiptera), the front pair of which is hardened to form protective coverings (hemi-elytra) for the rear pair (Fig. 3.21). They measure up to 4cm long; both sexes feed exclusively on blood. Most species belonging to the subfamily Triatominae (family Reduviidae) occur in South, Central and the southern part of North America, but a few are found in Asia.

Life cycle

All Hemiptera have five wingless immature stages (nymphs) in their life cycle, the fifth of which moults to form the adult. The life cycle takes 4–48 months for completion, depending on the temperature and the species. All stages (nymphs and adults) feed only on blood, so all can act as vectors of trypanosomes; they imbibe considerable quantities of blood, 100–300mg when adult.

The eggs are laid in cracks and crevices in mud-walled houses and furniture or in the nests or burrows of the mammals or birds on which the bugs feed. Adults in captivity may live for a year or more; in nature, most probably die before this.

Species

Within the subfamily Triatominae, which includes the vectors of *Trypanosoma cruzi*, there are 14 genera and around 111 species, over 90 of which have been found to be naturally infected with trypanosomes morphologically indistinguishable from *T. cruzi*, and presumably infective to human beings. Only the 10 or so species which come into close contact with people are important vectors of human infection, and most of these species belong to the genera *Panstrongylus*, *Rhodnius* and *Triatoma*.

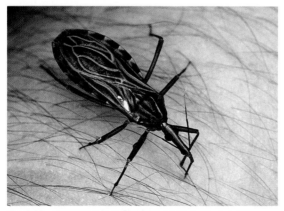

Fig. 3.21 Triatomine bug, *Rhodnius prolixus*. Courtesy of C J Scofield.

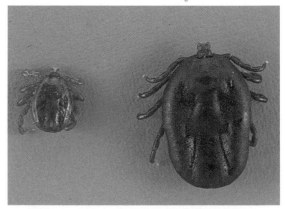

Fig. 3.22 Adult male (left) and female (right) of a hard tick (*Dermacentor*). The capitulum or 'false head' is visible from above, while almost the entire dorsal surface is covered by a hard shield.

Many species are sylvatic, that is, they live mainly in trees and forests, but some, notably *Triatoma infestans* and *Panstrongylus megistus*, have become domestic and inhabit houses and, in the case of *P. megistus*, palms and other trees growing around houses. *Rhodnius prolixus* normally lives in peri-domestic palm trees, but is introduced to houses when the palm leaves are used for thatch. These three species are therefore important vectors of human Chagas' disease.

Control

The best method of controlling the vector bug populations is the provision of housing of a relatively high standard, for example, built of brick or concrete blocks rather than mud, which cracks when it dries and provides ideal niches for bugs to colonize, and roofed with corrugated iron or similar materials rather than thatch. Household cleanliness is also important, to remove bugs and eggs from furniture etc. Insecticidal spraying of houses is effective in removing domestic species of bugs, benzene hexachloride being one of the more effective insecticides. Control of sylvatic bugs is well-nigh impossible.

BEDBUGS

Adult bedbugs of the order Hemiptera, family Cimicidae, are oval, wingless insects, about 4–5mm long and flattened dorsoventrally. Both sexes take blood

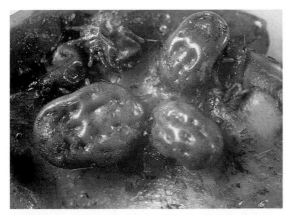

Fig. 3.23 Specimens of a soft tick (*Otobius*). The integument is tough and rubbery and without a hard dorsal shield. The capitulum is not visible from above.

meals at night and then retreat to their hiding places in crevices in beds, furniture and walls of houses.

Life cycle

Females lay one or two eggs a day which hatch in 4 days above 27°C but take several weeks at 17°C. There are 5 nymphal stages, each of which is blood-feeding, and maturity is reached in 5 to many weeks depending on temperature and availability of hosts.

Although the bites of bedbugs may cause considerable irritation, they are not known to be responsible for transmitting any disease, although suspected of transmitting hepatitis B.

Species

There are two species which commonly feed on man: *Cimex lectularius* in temperate regions and *C. hemipterus* which is more restricted to the tropics.

Control

Beds, bedclothes, furniture, floors and walls of infested houses should be sprayed with insecticide. Fogging can be used.

TICKS

Ticks together with mites belong to the class Arachnida. Members have 4 pairs of legs and a body divided into two regions in some mites, or undivided in ticks. Ticks are divided into two families, the Ixodiidae containing the hard ticks and the Argasidae or soft ticks.

Hard ticks have a hard shield-shaped plate, the scutum, which covers the anterior part of the dorsal surface in the female, or the whole surface in the male. The mouthparts are visible from above and have a pair of cutting and piercing chelicerae (Fig. 3.22). These are embedded in the host and the mouthparts form a tubular food channel through which blood is taken up and saliva injected.

Soft ticks have a folded cuticle without a dorsal plate and the mouthparts cannot be seen from above (Fig. 3.23). Hard ticks feed on one host for many days while soft ticks typically live in the nest or burrow and take many shorter feeds; neither group is very host specific.

The wounds made by ticks often become infected, particularly if the ticks are forcibly removed leaving their mouthparts embedded in the skin. Tick paralysis can also follow the bites of many species of hard ticks if they are located at the back of the neck. This starts around 2 days after a rapidly engorging female tick attaches, first paralysing the legs, then the arms and finally the thorax and throat. Death can result from respiratory failure, unless the tick is removed. The effect appears to be caused by neurotoxins in the tick saliva.

Life cycle

After feeding, the impregnated female drops off and lays a brown mass of eggs on the ground. The larvae are 6-legged and need to find a passing animal and feed on blood before dropping off to develop into a nymph which repeats the process and develops into a female or male adult. The same or different species of mammals may serve as hosts for the several stages.

Species

Many tick species, as well as being parasitic in themselves, can also transmit diseases of medical and veterinary importance, as shown in Fig. 3.24.

The most medically important genus of soft tick is *Ornithodorus*, commonly found in most warm parts of the world. Other genera sometimes found on man are *Argas* and *Otobius*.

Genera of hard ticks of medical importance include *Ixodes, Hyalomma, Amblyomma, Dermacentor, Rhipicephalus* and *Haemaphysalis* while the genus *Boophilus* is of great veterinary importance.

Control

A tick should be removed gently to avoid leaving its mouthparts behind. The process can be aided by smearing its abdomen with oil or fat, or by dabbing with an anaesthetic such as chloroform.

Houses infested with soft ticks can be sprayed with various insecticides such as malathion, carbaryl or organophosphorous compounds, paying particular attention to cracks in walls and furniture.

SCABIES MITES

Scabies mites (*Sarcoptes scabei*) have a worldwide distribution and, although they do not transmit any disease, they can cause intense itching.

tick	distribution	disease	causative organism	
Ornithodorus	Africa, Mediterranean	Endemic relapsing fever	Spirochaetes:	*Borrelia duttoni*
	North America, USSR			*Borrelia* spp.
Hard & Soft Ticks (*Dermacentor*)	North America, Europe, Japan	Tularaemia	Bacteria:	*Pasteurella tularensis*
	North & South America	American spotted fever	Rickettsias:	*R. rickettsii*
	Mediterranean	Boutonneuse fever	Rickettsias:	*R. conorii*
	Africa, Asia, Australia	Tick typhus	Rickettsias:	*R. conorii*
	Probably worldwide	Q fever	Rickettsias:	*R. australis* *Coxiella burneti*
Hard Ticks	Worldwide on animals	Piroplasmosis	Protozoa:	*Babesia*
	Africa & Asia	Piroplasmosis of livestock Anaplasmosis of sheep & cattle	Protozoa: Protozoa:	*Theileria* *Anaplasma*
(*Ixodes*)	Siberia	Encephalitis	Viruses	
	Europe	Louping ill of sheep	Viruses	
Hard & Soft Ticks (*Dermacentor*)	Western USA	Colorado tick fever	Viruses	

Fig. 3.24 Ticks as disease vectors.

Female mites measure 0.3–0.45mm, just visible to the naked eye, while males are about half as big. Adults have four pairs of legs, the first two ending in sucker-like organs, and pincer-like mouthparts (Fig. 3.25).

Epidemics of scabies usually occur in 20–30 year cycles or in times of war or famine but mites may be common at all times in very poor communities with inadequate washing facilities. The scabies itch usually takes 6–8 weeks to appear after first infection when the patient becomes sensitized, and is characteristically nocturnal. Septic pustules can develop after scratching if hygiene is poor. Sometimes there is a rash on the buttocks, waist, axillae, wrists and ankles, caused by a cell-mediated reaction. In immunodepressed individuals, there may be great multiplication of mites with extensive thickening and crusting of the skin which comes to resemble cornflakes.

The localization of the rash is characteristic but a definite diagnosis is made by smearing black ink on to the suspected areas and wiping excess away – the burrows will show up as black lines; or by making skin scrapings and examining microscopically for the presence of mites.

Life cycle

Impregnated females excavate burrows in the epidermis, especially where the skin is thin and wrinkled such as between the fingers and toes, axillae, genitals etc. These burrows appear as a tortuous grey line, up to 20mm in length, in dark-skinned people appearing as a pale line, and filled with excrement and eggs. Eggs hatch in 3–5 days and larvae emerge; if female, they enter a hair follicle and form moulting pockets where the young adult females are fertilized.

It is not completely clear how the mites are transmitted, although it does appear that prolonged close physical contact (over 15 minutes) is necessary for mature females to burrow from one skin to another, and infection is often familial.

Species

Sarcoptes scabei or other species in domestic animals cause the disease of sarcoptic mange but the latter do not become permanently established on man.

Treatment

Treatment of the whole body from the neck down with 1 per cent malathion or gamma benzene hexachloride, or crotamiton for infants, is recommended, while benzyl benzoate is also effective and is very cheap, although painful on broken skin. Topical steroids must not be used. If possible a whole family should be treated.

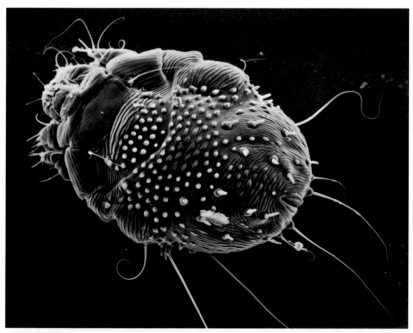

Fig. 3.25 Scanning electron micrograph of a scabies mite (*Sarcoptes*) removed from a burrow in the skin. They are minute and can be identified by the 8 short stumpy legs and numerous peg-like structures on the dorsal surface.

MITES: TROMBICULID SPECIES

Common names: chiggers, harvest mites, red bugs.

Different species, all formerly placed in one genus, *Trombicula*, occur in most parts of the world. The adults are bright red in colour and about 1mm long.

These mites can cause intense itching and irritation, due to sensitization to their saliva, after walking through long grass or scrub.

Life cycle
Eggs are laid on the ground and on leaves of grass, and the six-legged larvae which hatch out lay in wait for any passing mammal. They sink their sawed chelicerae into the skin, inject saliva and feed on tissue fluids until engorged, then drop off. They develop into nymphs and then adults, neither of which bite man or animals.

Species
In Asia, *Leptotrombidium* species can transmit *Rickettsia tsutsugamushi*, the cause of scrub typhus. The larvae bite only one host so there is no direct transmission of the rickettsia. A larva bites an infected individual and passes on the rickettsia taken up to its offspring (transovarial transmission). Large numbers of mites often occupy small 'islands' of vegetation in cleared forest areas which harbour numerous rodent hosts.

There are several other genera of mites which can occasionally cause irritation but the only common one is *Demodex folliculorum*, the hair follicle mite, which is present in a high proportion of adults but only rarely causes adverse effects such as dermatitis or acne.

4. DIAGNOSTIC TECHNIQUES

The aim of this chapter is not to give details of techniques but to indicate those which may be used. The reader can then obtain further practical details from the books listed in the further reading section.

PARASITOLOGICAL TECHNIQUES USING FAECES

Specimens for examination must be fresh, that is, promptly collected and uncontaminated by other material, such as soil, or free-living coprozoic protozoa and nematode larvae may colonize them and cause difficulty in diagnosis. If specimens are kept too long, any protozoan trophozoites present will die; if specimens cannot be examined immediately, they should be stored in closed containers and refrigerated at 4°C, if possible. If there is likely to be a long delay, specimens may be preserved in either of the following (though these kill trophozoites):

- formol-saline; one volume of formalin
(10 per cent aq. HCHO)
9 volumes of saline
(0.9 per cent aq. NaCl)

- MIF fixative; 250ml distilled water
200ml tincture of merthiolate
25ml formaldehyde
5ml glycerol
15 parts of Lugol's iodine solution
(5 per cent iodine in 10 per cent potassium iodide)

Faeces can be examined microscopically, either directly or after cultivation. Care must be taken not to contaminate fingers and accidentally ingest cysts or eggs when examining fresh faeces, as these may be infective; all material must be safely disposed of, either into suitable disinfectant (such as Chloros, Lysol) or into closed containers for subsequent incineration or autoclaving.

Direct examination

Three preparations should be made, if possible, by mixing a small portion (pin head size) with a swab-stick or matchstick in:

- (a) 0.9 per cent saline; this is the least essential,

and should be made only if the material is really fresh (warm), as its main purpose is to find any protozoan trophozoites and *Strongyloides* larvae, though of course cysts and helminths eggs may also be seen.

- (b) 1 per cent aqueous eosin solution. If it is not too thick, living protozoal cysts or helminth eggs stand out as unstained, white objects against a reddish-pink background; any which are seen should be examined at about ×400 magnification.

- (c) iodine solution (4 per cent KI plus 2 per cent I_2 in distilled water). This preparation should be examined last, when the microscopist will have some idea of what cysts or eggs are present, as a result of prior examination of specimens (a) or (b), or both, and any cysts or eggs present should be examined at about ×400 (and for protozoal cysts at about ×1000 if necessary, using an oil-immersion objective).

A modified Kato thick smear method can be used for helminth eggs. A roughly 50mg faecal sample (sieved if necessary) is placed on a microscope slide and covered with a large cover-slip made of cellophane (such as from a cigarette packet) which has been soaked in 1 part ethanediol, 1 part formalin and 2

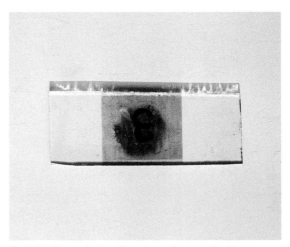

Fig. 4.1 Kato technique. Faecal sample covered with cellophane coverslip and becoming transparent. Courtesy of Dr K Kato.

parts of saturated saline; a few drops of 3 per cent aqueous malachite green can also be added to make the transparent eggs stand out better (Fig. 4.1). The slide is turned over and pressed on to thick filter paper and then examined when the faeces has cleared.

Concentration

Scanty cysts or eggs can be made easier to find by concentrating them before making specimens. Concentration techniques depend on differences in density between cysts and eggs, and most of the faecal debris. One common technique involves flotation of the faecal specimen in aqueous zinc sulphate solution; cysts and eggs rise to the surface. Another, better, method depends on centrifugation of the specimen, after emulsification in a mixture of formol-saline and ether, followed by examination of half of the deposit after staining with iodine and half after mixing with Sargeaunt's stain, useful for identifying protozoal cysts, as it stains both nuclei and chromatoid bodies (if present).

Cultivation

Another method of revealing the presence of very sparse cysts of *Entamoeba histolytica* or *Balantidium coli* is to inoculate some faeces into a tube of suitable

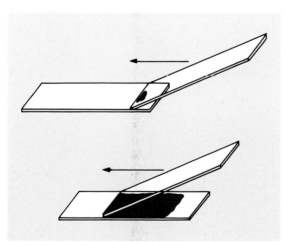

Fig. 4.2 Preparation of a thin blood film.

culture medium, incubate it at 37°C and examine a drop microscopically to detect the presence of trophozoites which may have emerged from scanty cysts. A commonly used medium is Dobell and Laidlow's HSre, which consists of a slant of horse serum coagulated by heat and covered with a solution of egg albumen in Ringer's saline.

Cultivation techniques can also be used for revealing first stage *Strongyloides* larvae in faeces. In the Harada–Mori method around half a gram of faeces is smeared along a strip of filter paper leaving 5cm clear at the bottom. This is placed in a test tube containing 7ml of distilled water and the covered test tube left for 4 days at 28°C. The longer and more easily seen infective larvae will be in the water at the bottom and can be examined microscopically after preserving with formalin.

PARASITOLOGICAL TECHNIQUES USING BLOOD

Blood, like faeces, can be examined for parasites (protozoa or microfilariae), either directly or after concentration, or by cultivation. Precautions to avoid accidental infection of the examiner must be strictly observed; gloves should be worn when handling fresh blood and great care taken to avoid accidental piercing of gloves and skin with blood lancets, needles and so on. Any wound must be *immediately* washed with 70 per cent alcohol. Materials must be safely disposed of by the methods used for faeces.

Direct examination

A drop of blood is obtained by pricking a fingertip (or with babies, an earlobe or foot) with a sterile disposable lancet, after sterilizing the skin with alcohol and allowing it to dry. (A fresh sterile lancet *must* be used for each person, or infections may be transferred; used lancets must be disposed of *immediately* into disinfectant or closed container.)

The drop is then used to make thin or thick blood films (or both). A thin film is made by depositing a small drop of blood at one end of a clean microscope slide and spreading out into a layer, one cell thick, by pushing with the edge of another slide held at 45° to the first (Fig. 4.2). For a thick film, a larger drop (of about 20mm^3) is placed on the slide and gently spread out thinly enough for the numbers of a wrist-watch to be just visible through it (Fig. 4.3).

After thorough drying, thin films (*not* thick films) are fixed by brief immersion in methanol, and both types of film can then be stained with Giemsa's, Wright's or Leishman's stains. Thick films can also be stained with Field's stain (for malaria parasites) or with haematoxylin (for microfilariae; Giemsa's and Leishman's stains do not stain all microfilarial sheaths). The staining of trypanosomes in thick films by Giemsa's stain is improved by brief (1 second) prior immersion in 0.5 per cent aq. methylene blue. For microfilariae it is necessary to dehaemoglobinize the thoroughly dried (24 hours) thick smear in distilled water first.

Thick films are, in effect, a simple concentration technique, but morphological details of protozoa are less well preserved and examination of thin films may be necessary for accurate specific diagnosis.

Concentration

Blood parasites can be simply concentrated by Woo's haematocrit centrifuge technique. Blood is collected (from a finger prick) into a heparinized microhaematocrit tube which is then centrifuged. Protozoa (trypanosomes and malaria-infected erythrocytes) and microfilariae collect at the interface between packed erythrocytes and plasma. Trypanosomes and microfilariae can be visualized there by microscopical examination ($\times 100$ or $\times 400$) through the wall of the tube, preferably after mounting it on a slide in a small pool of immersion oil. Malaria parasites can be seen by making a thick or thin film of the interface layer, by scoring the tube at this point with a diamond, breaking it and expelling a drop of the topmost layer of erythrocytes on to a slide (gloves must be worn and all other precautions be strictly adhered to during this process: see above).

For microfilariae, blood can be filtered through a $5\mu m$ pore size nuclepore membrane filter attached to a 10ml hypodermic syringe and the dried membrane stained and examined microscopically.

Cultivation

Blood collected by venepuncture into a heparinized syringe can be used to inoculate suitable culture media to facilitate the finding of very scarce *Leishmania* or trypanosomes. Material collected by aseptic puncture of the periphery of a lesion of suspected cutaneous leishmaniasis, or bone marrow collected by sternal puncture from suspected cases of visceral leishmaniasis, can be treated similarly.

Trypanosoma cruzi and *Leishmania* spp. will usually grow in NNN or 4N media (based on blood, and simple or nutrient agar respectively); for *T. brucei*, more complex media (such as Weinman's) are required. Cultures are incubated at 24–28°C and examined (with sterile precautions) weekly, for up to 4 weeks, for the presence of motile flagellates.

Xenodiagnosis

This technique is used for the diagnosis of Chagas' disease. Uninfected laboratory-reared bugs are allowed to feed on the suspect patient, and afterwards bug faeces (or hind-gut contents) are examined for the presence of motile flagellates, about 4 weeks later.

IMMUNODIAGNOSTIC TECHNIQUES

Parasites have complex macromolecules on their surface or in their secretions and excretions. These antigens are recognized as foreign by specific antibody molecules in man which bind to them. Most immunodiagnostic tests make use of the presence of antibodies in a blood sample from an infected person which will react with an antigen preparation from the parasite in such a way that results can be observed visually. The body can produce millions of different antibodies each of which will bind to a specific part of an antigen only (an epitope).

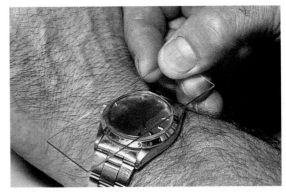

Fig. 4.3 A thick blood film of the correct size and thickness. Sometimes both thin and thick films are placed on the same microscope slide.

Most of the techniqes in use for the immuno-diagnosis of parasites are based on those first described for viruses and bacteria although there are some special techniques which rely on reactions against whole parasites or life cycle stages (see pages 23, 31 and 65).

It is possible to review the standard tests only in the briefest outline; for further details the further reading list should be consulted. A summary of immunodiagnostic techniques used in parasitic infections is given in Fig. 4.4.

Intradermal

Intradermal or skin tests involve a type I hypersensitivity reaction (p.149) following the injection of a small amount of parasite antigen into the skin causing a red itchy lump (weal and flare) in sensitized individuals 30 minutes later (Fig. 2.53). The test is

Fig. 4.4 Summary of immuno-diagnostic techniques used in parasitic infections.

	Page reference	Immuno-electrophoresis	Counter-electrophoresis	Agglutination	Complement fixation	Immunofluorescence	ELISA
Comparative Sensitivity		++	++	+++	+++	+++	+++
Speed		1 day	3hrs	2hrs	2hrs	2hrs	4hrs
Malaria	19	●	●	●		○	○
Toxoplasmosis*	23			○	●	○	●
African trypanosomiasis	31			○	●	●	●
Chagas' disease*	35		●	●	●	●	●
Leishmaniasis	39		●			●	●
Amoebiasis	47	●	●	●	●	●	●
Schistosomiasis	65	●	●	●		●	○
Fascioliasis*	73	●	○	●	○		●
Cysticercosis*	84	●	●	●	●	●	○
Echinococcosis*	88	●	○	○		●	○
Lymphatic filariasis	106	●	●	●		●	●
Onchocerciasis	111	●		●		●	●
Trichinosis*	114	●	●	○	●	●	○
Toxocariasis*	116	●		●		●	○
Strongyloidiasis	96			●	●	●	●

● techniques sometimes used
○ standard techniques most widely used
* infections for which immunodiagnosis is most useful

not now much used since it is very non-specific and is positive for several years after parasites have vanished.

Precipitation

Precipitation tests include the standard double diffusion reaction in gels (Ouchterlony test) and recent modifications. In immunoelectrophoresis a pH is chosen so that antigens are first separated by an electric current on the basis of their positive or negative charge before being visualized by a precipitation reaction with antibody. In countercurrent immunoelectrophoresis (CIE) a current is passed across the gel to move negatively charged antigen and positively charged antibody towards each other, increasing the sensitivity by up to 20 fold.

Haemagglutination

Haemagglutination (HA and Indirect HA) tests rely on antibody binding to antigen coated on red blood cells and agglutinating them. By using doubling dilutions of serum this and all the subsequently described tests can give quantitative assays of antibody. Modifications have used latex or bentonite particles instead of red blood cells (pp.88 and 114).

Complement fixation

In the complement fixation (CF) test, a test antiserum is titrated in doubling dilutions and a fixed amount of antigen added to each. Then complement (p.144) is added at a concentration just sufficient to lyse red cells which are added next. If specific antibodies are present in the original serum they form complexes with the antigen and fix the complement so the red cells will not lyse.

Indirect immunofluorescence

The indirect immunofluorescence test (IFAT) is very useful for detecting antibodies to tissue and cellular antigens. Protozoa in smears or cryostat sections of

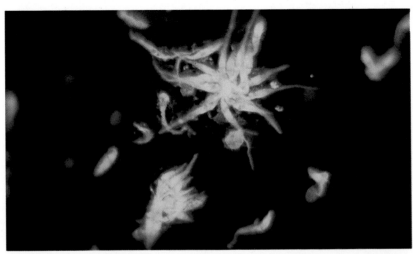

Fig. 4.5 IFAT. Slide coated with culture of *Trypanosoma cruzi*, the surface of which appears light green under the fluorescence microscope. This is a positive result showing that the test serum, at the particular dilution used, contained antibodies to this organism. Courtesy of Dr A Voller.

helminths on microscope slides are used as the antigen and doubling dilutions of serum added. After washing, a fluorescein-bound anti-human immunoglobulin conjugate (ligand) is added and unbound reagent then washed off. The preparation is examined under a fluorescence microscope and fluoresces only where the antibody has bound to the antigen and the conjugate has in turn bound to the globulin portion of the antibody (Fig. 4.5).

Enzyme Linked Immunosorbent Assay

The Enzyme Linked Immunosorbent Assay (ELISA) involves incubating the antigen on plastic micro plates or in tubes. Small quantities become adsorbed on to the plastic surface. The serially diluted serum is added after washing with saline then, with further washes, anti-human immunoglobulin labelled with an enzyme, often peroxidase (ligand), is incubated on the plates or in the tubes, followed by a substrate which changes colour after enzyme degradation. The intensity of colour is proportional to antibody concentration.

ELISA is extremely sensitive and a large number of tests can be performed automatically in a short time using minute quantities of antigen. The test can use dried spots of finger-prick blood on filter paper and, once suitable reagents have been made, can be employed under field conditions. This technique will clearly become a routine method of diagnosing many parasitic infections in the near future.

Radioimmunoassay

Radioimmunoassay (RIA) uses a similar procedure to ELISA except that the ligand is radiolabelled and radioactivity is measured in a gamma counter. The radioallergosorbent test (RAST) is a radioimmunoassay which measures antigen-specific IgE (see p. 146) present in serum only in small quantities, by using radiolabelled anti-IgE antibody.

Monoclonal antibodies and recombinant DNA

One of the major restraints to the wide use of immunodiagnostic tests in the diagnosis of parasitic diseases (apart from the cost of some of the equipment needed) is the difficulty of obtaining specific antigens which do not cross-react. Also, antibodies may remain in the serum long after the parasite has disappeared. A new approach is the detection of antigen rather than antibody (for instance infections with *Entamoeba* or *Giardia* can already be detected by immunological identification of parasite antigen in the faeces).

The production of specific antigenic determinants in large quantities has been greatly aided by monoclonal antibody and recombinant DNA techniques. In the former, a parasite antigen is injected into a mouse, a culture of antibody producing B cells from the spleen removed and fused with 'immortal' tumour cells and the remaining hybridoma cells cultured and tested for the desired antibody production (by ELISA or RIA). Clones of cells can be produced from a single isolated cell removed and grown in cultures to express large quantities of a single (monoclonal) antibody.

Recombinant DNA techniques depend on the use of a battery of enzymes to manipulate isolated DNA from an organism and to split it into fragments at highly specific sites by the use of other enzymes (restriction endonucleases) derived from microorganisms, each of which recognizes a precise sequence of nucleotides.

Gene length fragments of DNA are cloned in either bacteriophage or plasmid vectors (rings of extranuclear DNA usually from *Escherichia coli*) on a phage plate in order to replicate the fragments and build up a gene library. To identify the location of specific genes expressed as proteins it is necessary to blot the plate with a nitrocellulose overlay containing a radio-labelled antibody probe. The required portion of the phage plate is removed and grown further. In addition to their use in immunodiagnosis, gene cloning techniques are also being used for differentiation of morphologically indistinguishable strains of parasites.

In addition to their value in immunodiagnosis, it has been possible using these techniques to recognize and sometimes synthesize antigens which elicit protective immune responses and thus could be the basis for development of anti-parasite vaccines. Often these antigens are stage specific, so that for malaria there are projected sporozoite, merozoite, schizont and gametocyte vaccines.

For the clinical diagnosis of most parasitic diseases, immunodiagnostic techniques take second place to parasitological. However, for infections in which stages are not present in faeces or blood or in which early diagnosis is important, they are often necessary (see Fig. 4.4). In addition, immunodiagnostic tests can be of epidemiological importance in establishing endemicity and in assessing changes in transmission during or after control schemes.

5. IMMUNOLOGY AND IMMUNOPATHOLOGY

INTRODUCTION

This is a rapidly developing and increasingly complex field of study and it is only possible here to give what must be a very brief and superficial resumé of basic immunological principles.

Immunity can be either innate or acquired. Innate immunity, or natural resistance, can be manifested in a variety of ways:

• the skin can protect against non-human species of schistosomes and hookworms;

• cysts or eggs ingested may not encounter the right conditions in the intestine for hatching;

• factors in human serum can destroy some strains of *Trypanosoma brucei* or factors on, or absent from,

red blood corpuscles prevent the entry of merozoites of *Plasmodium vivax* (presence of the Duffy blood group antigen absent in West Africans appears to be essential for their attachment and penetration).

If an organism does succeed in entering the tissues of the body it encounters various types of phagocytic cells (monocytes/macrophages, amine containing cells comprising mast cells and basophils, and granulocytes including neutrophils and eosinophils) all derived from bone marrow stem cells. In addition there is a complex of around 20 serum proteins, mostly proteinases, known as complement. Complement becomes activated by the surface of foreign organisms (and in acquired immunity also by antigen–antibody complexes in the classical pathway) and amplified by a cascading sequence of enzymatically

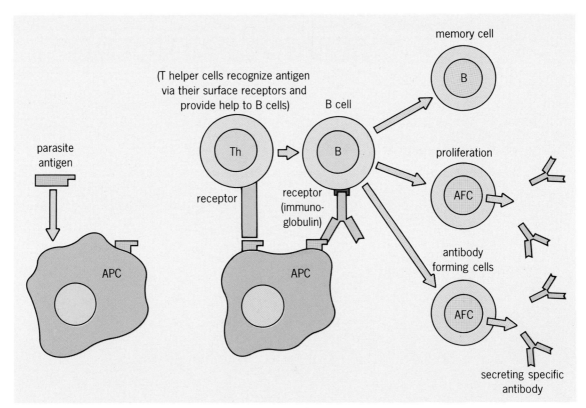

Fig. 5.1 Antibody response to antigen. APC = antigen presenting cell (in skin known as Langerhan's cell).

controlled processes giving forms (such as C_3) which are biologically active (for example releasing histamine and lysing cell membranes) by the alternative pathway. Components also promote the adherence of macrophages and chemoattraction of eosinophils and neutrophils.

Host genetic factors are of great importance in determining resistance to parasites. The ability to respond to particular antigens can be genetically determined and the genes responsible are associated with a particular region of one chromosome (number 6 in man) known as the major histocompatibility complex (MHC). Immune response genes are associated with the MHC and can be very specific; in mice it has been shown that substitution of a single amino acid can affect responsiveness.

In addition to the host's innate defences there is a complex interacting array of acquired mechanisms which are also activated by parasite invasion.

As well as the phagocytic cells and complement there is another group of cells derived from bone marrow which is an essential component of the immune system, the lymphocytes. There are two classes of lymphoid cells, T cells which develop in the thymus and are involved primarily with cell-mediated immune responses and with helper functions, and B cells which develop in the bone marrow and are associated with antibody-mediated processes. Both T and B cells carry receptors capable of combining with an antigenic epitope and, following stimulation by a specific antigen, of producing a clone of cells having receptors specific for that antigen (Fig. 5.1).

Antibody produced by B cells can be one of 5 different types of immunoglobulin (Figs 5.2 & 5.3). Antibodies combine with antigens and if the latter are soluble their toxins are neutralized and enzymes inactivated and the complex formed can be phagocytosed.

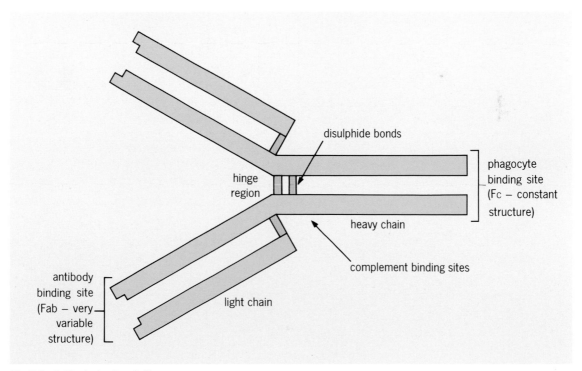

Fig. 5.2 Antibody structure (IgG).

The mechanisms by which antibodies attach to antigens on the cell surface of parasites or of cells containing protozoal parasites are shown in Fig. 5.4. In addition to antibody, many responses involve complement, and phagocytes have specific complement receptors. The adherence of macrophages and chemoattraction of eosinophils and neutrophils is promoted most powerfully when components of the complement cascade are activated by antibody.

The numbers of the following immune responses to parasites correspond to Fig. 5.4:

1 Complement comes in contact with the antigen surface and is activated by the non-antibody mediated alternative pathway. Phagocytes attach by complement receptors. Activated macrophages and neutrophils produce cytotoxic oxygen metabolites while the granules of eosinophils also produce cytotoxic substances.

2 IgG or IgE bind to the antigen, and phagocytes attach by specific receptors (as can mast cells and basophils).

3 IgG binds to the antigens and fixes complement. Phagocytes attach by both IgG and complement receptors.

4 IgM binds to antigen, activates the complement cascade by the classical pathway, and attracted phagocytes attach by complement receptors. Unlike IgG and IgE, phagocytes do not bind to IgM.

5 Antibodies form immune complexes with soluble antigens diffusing out and eosinophils and macrophages are attracted and attach to the antibody by specific receptors.

6 Macrophages, which have been activated non-specifically by substances (lymphokines) produced by T cells specifically stimulated by soluble antigens presented to them by antigen presenting cells, are attracted to any antigen.

Helminths differ from most infectious agents as they have large body surfaces and cannot be phagocytosed. Cytotoxic T lymphocytes active against viruses and bacteria are usually ineffective and instead there are high IgE responses with an increase in the numbers of mast cells and particularly of eosinophils. Eosinophils attack parasite surfaces as well as removing histamine produced by mast cell degranulation which is also initiated by IgE. IgE can also activate macrophages to become cytotoxic (in a similar way to the more usual T cell activation of macrophages). Neutrophil attack by oxidative killing mechanisms (such as the release of hydrogen peroxide) mediated by both antibodies (usually IgG) and complement is particularly effective against the sheath of nematode larvae such as microfilariae.

Fig. 5.3 Antibody classes.

IgG – 70–75% of total antibody. In serum. Fixes complement.

IgM – 15–20% of total. In serum and can be secreted across mucous surfaces. Often first antibody produced in response to antigenic stimulation. 5 antibody molecules join to form polymer. Fixes complement.

IgE – Tiny amounts in serum and on surface of basophils and mast cells. Appears to be particularly important against helminths.

IgA – 15–20% of total. Found in seromucous secretions (saliva etc.).

IgD – 1%. Functions unknown.

EVASION AND SUPPRESSION OF HOST IMMUNE RESPONSES BY PARASITES

Site

Parasites which are intracellular, such as *Trypanosoma cruzi*, *Leishmania* spp. and intracellular stages of *Plasmodium* spp., are to some extent protected from the action of antibodies as are those that form cysts, such as *Toxoplasma gondii*, and larvae of *Taenia solium*, *Echinococcus granulosus* and *Trichinella spiralis*.

Parasites which live in macrophages such as *Toxoplasma gondii*, *Trypanosoma cruzi* and *Leishmania* spp.

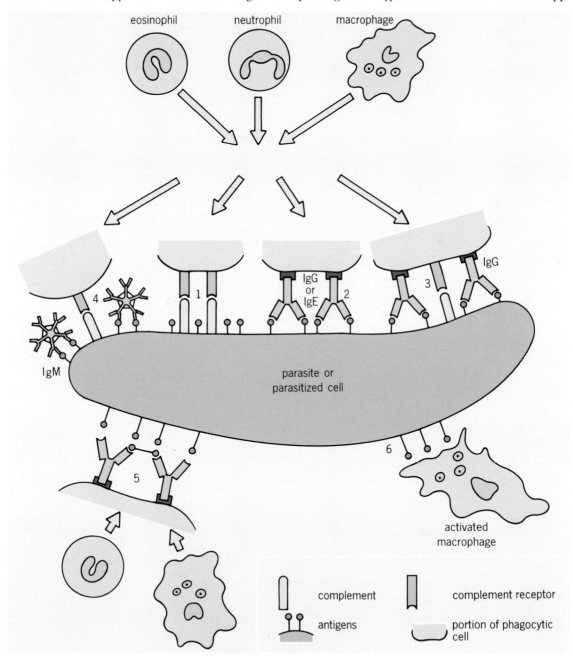

Fig. 5.4 The different types of protective responses of phagocytes to parasites or to cells containing parasites. Small parasites may be engulfed or the surface of larger ones attacked.

are able to avoid or inactivate the lysosomal enzymes and oxygen metabolites which are the cells' weapons of offence against microbial organisms.

Avoidance of recognition

Cyclical variation of the surface antigens by African trypanosomes was considered on page 28 and a similar process by some erythrocytic stages of *Plasmodium* on page 14.

Schistosomes are capable of masking their foreignness by acquiring a surface layer of host antigens which possibly protects them from antibody damage. This process is aided by rapid replacement of the surface tegument. It applies only to adult worms present in the blood vessels, not to new invading larvae (schistosomules); a process termed concomitant immunity, since the presence of adults continues to stimulate immune responses directed against new invasive stages.

Infection	Clinical manifestation	Type of reaction
Malaria	Nephrotic syndrome (*P. malariae*) Anaemia	III II
Chagas' disease	Megacolon; Myocarditis	II
Leishmaniasis	Spectrum of disease (Spleen and liver enlargement or skin lesions)	IV
African trypanosomiasis	Glomerulonephritis? Vasculitis	III
Ascariasis	Urticaria; Asthma	I
Schistosomiasis	Swimmer's itch due to cercariae Katayama fever due to young schistosomes Granulomas caused by eggs Glomerulonephritis caused by eggs	I, IV III IV III
Echinococcosis	Leakage of hydatid cyst with general anaphylaxis	I
Trichinosis	Inflammatory response to larvae in muscle	I
Lymphatic filariasis	Elephantiasis TPE	IV I
Onchocerciasis	Chronic skin lesions	III?
Tick bites and scabies	Inflammation at site of bite or mite tunnel	I, IV

Fig. 5.5 Hypersensitivity reactions responsible for clinical disease in parasitic infection.

Suppression of the immune response

Non-specific immunodepression is a feature of many parasitic infections and has been demonstrated for both antibody and cell-mediated responses. This sometimes results in an increase in the severity of any viral or bacterial infections also present. Many parasites produce large quantities of soluble antigens which can spread widely and have varied immuno-suppressive effects, such as:

- combining with antibody and preventing it from attaching to the parasite;

- blocking the action of effector cells which are inhibited by circulating antibody–antigen complexes;

- inducing B or T cell tolerance either by blocking antibody forming cells or by depleting the stock of mature antigen specific lymphocytes (clonal exhaustion);

- activating specific suppressor cells (T cells or macrophages);

- initiating polyclonal activation. African trypanosomes for example accelerate the proliferation of B lymphocytes (probably causing the high serum concentrations of IgM and IgG typical of this infection) which can lead to general depletion of antigen-reactive B cells.

Leishmania is able to stimulate specific T suppressor cells which depress T cell reactivity and reduce the protective cell-mediated response, the host's main defence against this organism. Probably many more mechanisms of this type await discovery.

IMMUNOPATHOLOGY

During the primary immune response to any infectious agent specific memory B and T cells are generated in the body which enable the immune system to respond more rapidly to reinvasion by the same agent. While this acquired resistance response is aimed at overcoming the agent, in some parasitic diseases in particular (perhaps because of the large size of the agents) the response to the secondary infection can actually contribute to the pathology of the disease. These inappropriate reactions are termed hypersensitivity which was divided by Coombs and Gell in 1963 into four types. The clinical manifestations due to these reactions are summarized in Fig. 5.5

Despite these subdivisions, however, it is likely that in all parasitic diseases more than one mechanism is involved, possibly at the same time, but often there is a sequence of reactions and associated clinical manifestations at different stages of infection. It must not be thought that these reactions are entirely deleterious; for instance, if the granuloma did not form around schistosome eggs (see type IV reactions below), toxic products from the eggs would diffuse out and cause more widespread liver damage.

The four types of hypersensitivity reaction are outlined below.

Type I reaction (immediate hypersensitivity or anaphylaxis)

This is initiated by an allergen (such as pollen) or a parasite antigen reacting with mast cells or basophils (and probably other cells) which have been sensitized by antibody (IgE) and leads to degranulation and the release of vasoactive amines and other mediators of inflammation. However, the reaction appears to be of benefit in the expulsion of intestinal helminths.

Type II reaction (antibody dependent cytotoxicity)

Antibody (IgG or IgM) binds with antigens present on an individual's own cells (target cells) and can lead to complement-mediated lysis or to cytotoxic action by killer T cells.

Type III reaction (immune complex mediated damage)

Antibody–antigen complexes are formed as part of a normal host immune response and are eliminated by macrophages. However, under some circumstances such as chronic parasitic infections, complexes are deposited in tissues (particularly in the glomeruli of the kidney), complement is activated, and attracted granulocytes cause a tissue-damaging inflammatory response (for example nephritis due to *Plasmodium malariae* infection).

Type IV reactions
(delayed or cell-mediated hypersensitivity)

Antigen sensitized T cells release lymphokines (agents which activate and attract macrophages) and induce a capsule of inflammatory cells when the antigen is met again; if it cannot be cleared because the antigenic stimulation continues in chronic infections, as with schistosome eggs in the liver, a granuloma is produced and eventually fibrosis ensues (Fig. 5.6). Antibody is not involved.

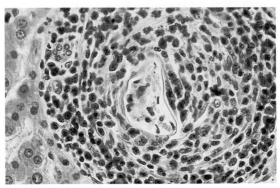 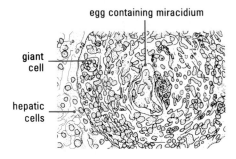

Fig. 5.6   Schistosome egg granuloma in the liver. A mixed leucocytic response walls off the egg.

APPENDICES

SUMMARY OF THE HABITAT AND PATHOLOGICAL EFFECTS OF PARASITES WITHIN THE BODY

In the main part of this book we have dealt with the various parasites in taxonomic order. However, from the point of view of comparative study, and also as a form of summary, the following appendices are included indicating which organs the parasites inhabit and what, if any, are their major pathological effects on those organs. For convenience and simplicity, we have divided the organ systems into 3 groups:

1) brain and central nervous system, lungs, heart, liver, spleen, pancreas and kidneys;

2) intestinal and urogenital systems;

3) eyes, blood, lymphatics, bone marrow, muscles, subcutaneous tissues and skin.

We have ignored organs through which parasites merely pass, and on which they have no detectable effect. The more important pathological effects are printed in bold type; such distinctions are, to some extent, arbitrary, and what is or is not significant may differ from individual to individual, or from parasite strain to parasite strain. This summary presentation should be regarded as giving only the broad outlines of the parasites' behaviour. For the sake of completeness, some parasites which are only occasionally found in humans are included, even though they are not mentioned further in the text. Rare human parasites are marked with an asterisk, as are uncommon sites or uncommon effects of the more common parasites.

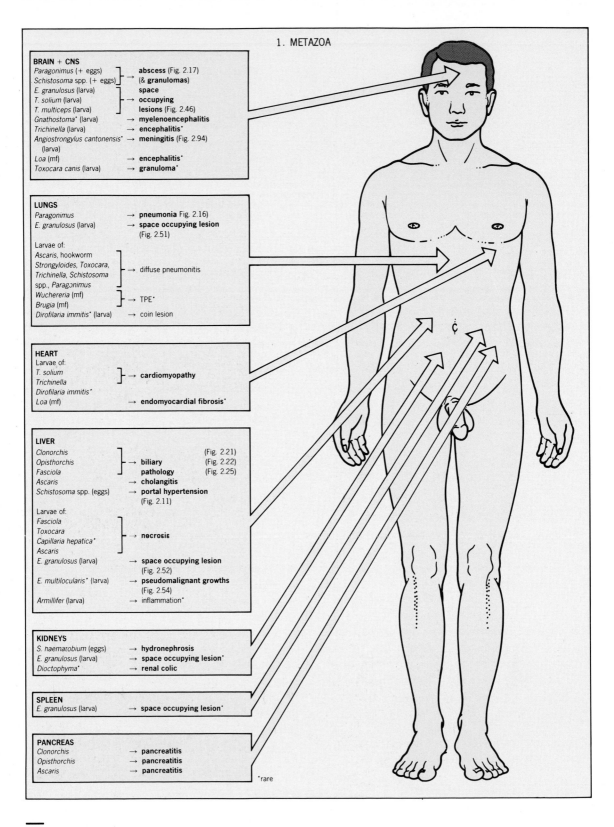

1. METAZOA

BRAIN + CNS
Paragonimus (+ eggs) → **abscess** (Fig. 2.17)
Schistosoma spp. (+ eggs) **(& granulomas)**
E. granulosus (larva) → **space**
T. solium (larva) → **occupying**
T. multiceps (larva) **lesions** (Fig. 2.46)
*Gnathostoma** (larva) → **myelenoencephalitis**
Trichinella (larva) → **encephalitis***
*Angiostrongylus cantonensis** → **meningitis** (Fig. 2.94)
  (larva)
Loa (mf) → **encephalitis***
Toxocara canis (larva) → **granuloma***

LUNGS
Paragonimus → **pneumonia** Fig. 2.16)
E. granulosus (larva) → **space occupying lesion**
  (Fig. 2.51)

Larvae of:
Ascaris, hookworm
Strongyloides, Toxocara, → diffuse pneumonitis
Trichinella, Schistosoma
spp., *Paragonimus*
Wuchereria (mf) → TPE*
Brugia (mf)
*Dirofilaria immitis** (larva) → coin lesion

HEART
Larvae of:
T. solium → **cardiomyopathy**
Trichinella
*Dirofilaria immitis**
Loa (mf) → **endomyocardial fibrosis***

LIVER
Clonorchis (Fig. 2.21)
Opisthorchis → **biliary** (Fig. 2.22)
Fasciola **pathology** (Fig. 2.25)
Ascaris → **cholangitis**
Schistosoma spp. (eggs) → **portal hypertension**
  (Fig. 2.11)

Larvae of:
Fasciola
Toxocara
*Capillaria hepatica** → **necrosis**
Ascaris
E. granulosus (larva) → **space occupying lesion**
  (Fig. 2.52)
*E. multilocularis** (larva) → **pseudomalignant growths**
  (Fig. 2.54)
Armillifer (larva) → **inflammation***

KIDNEYS
S. haematobium (eggs) → **hydronephrosis**
E. granulosus (larva) → **space occupying lesion***
*Dioctophyma** → **renal colic**

SPLEEN
E. granulosus (larva) → **space occupying lesion***

PANCREAS
Clonorchis → **pancreatitis**
Opisthorchis → **pancreatitis**
Ascaris → **pancreatitis**

*rare

152

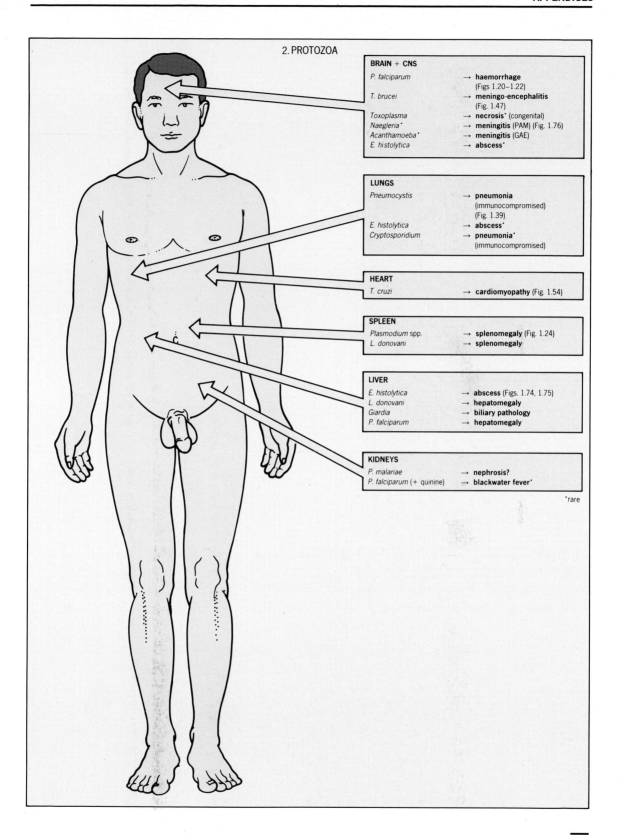

2. PROTOZOA

BRAIN + CNS

P. falciparum	→	**haemorrhage** (Figs 1.20–1.22)
T. brucei	→	**meningo-encephalitis** (Fig. 1.47)
Toxoplasma *	→	**necrosis** * (congenital)
Naegleria *	→	**meningitis** (PAM) (Fig. 1.76)
Acanthamoeba *	→	**meningitis** (GAE)
E. histolytica	→	**abscess** *

LUNGS

Pneumocystis	→	**pneumonia** (immunocompromised) (Fig. 1.39)
E. histolytica	→	**abscess** *
Cryptosporidium	→	**pneumonia** * (immunocompromised)

HEART

T. cruzi	→	**cardiomyopathy** (Fig. 1.54)

SPLEEN

Plasmodium spp.	→	**splenomegaly** (Fig. 1.24)
L. donovani	→	**splenomegaly**

LIVER

E. histolytica	→	**abscess** (Figs. 1.74, 1.75)
L. donovani	→	**hepatomegaly**
Giardia	→	**biliary pathology**
P. falciparum	→	**hepatomegaly**

KIDNEYS

P. malariae	→	**nephrosis?**
P. falciparum (+ quinine)	→	**blackwater fever** *

*rare

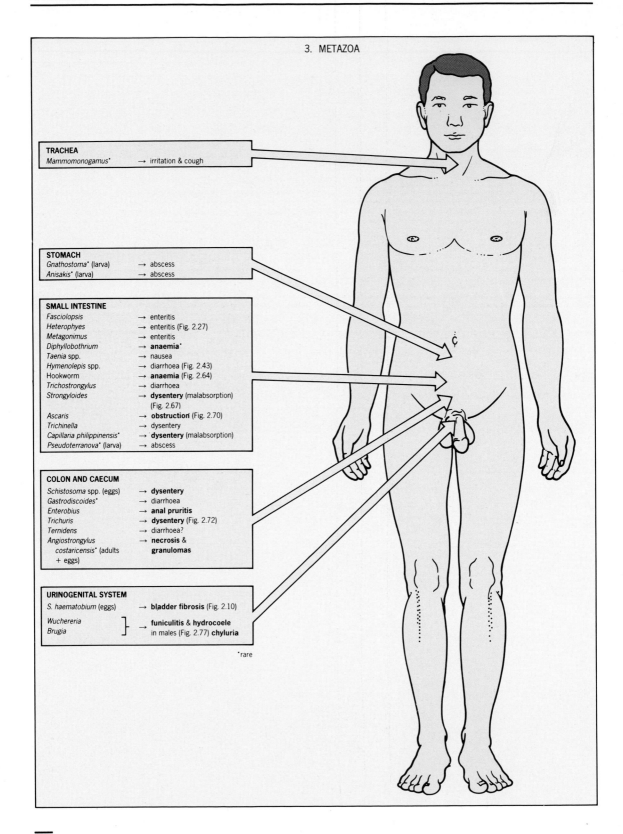

3. METAZOA

TRACHEA
*Mammomonogamus** → irritation & cough

STOMACH
*Gnathostoma** (larva) → abscess
*Anisakis** (larva) → abscess

SMALL INTESTINE
Fasciolopsis → enteritis
Heterophyes → enteritis (Fig. 2.27)
Metagonimus → enteritis
Diphyllobothrium → **anaemia***
Taenia spp. → nausea
Hymenolepis spp. → diarrhoea (Fig. 2.43)
Hookworm → **anaemia** (Fig. 2.64)
Trichostrongylus → diarrhoea
Strongyloides → **dysentery** (malabsorption) (Fig. 2.67)
Ascaris → **obstruction** (Fig. 2.70)
Trichinella → dysentery
*Capillaria philippinensis** → **dysentery** (malabsorption)
*Pseudoterranova** (larva) → abscess

COLON AND CAECUM
Schistosoma spp. (eggs) → **dysentery**
*Gastrodiscoides** → diarrhoea
Enterobius → **anal pruritis**
Trichuris → **dysentery** (Fig. 2.72)
Ternidens → diarrhoea?
Angiostrongylus → **necrosis** &
  *costaricensis** (adults **granulomas**
  + eggs)

URINOGENITAL SYSTEM
S. haematobium (eggs) → **bladder fibrosis** (Fig. 2.10)
Wuchereria
Brugia] → **funiculitis** & **hydrocoele** in males (Fig. 2.77) **chyluria**

*rare

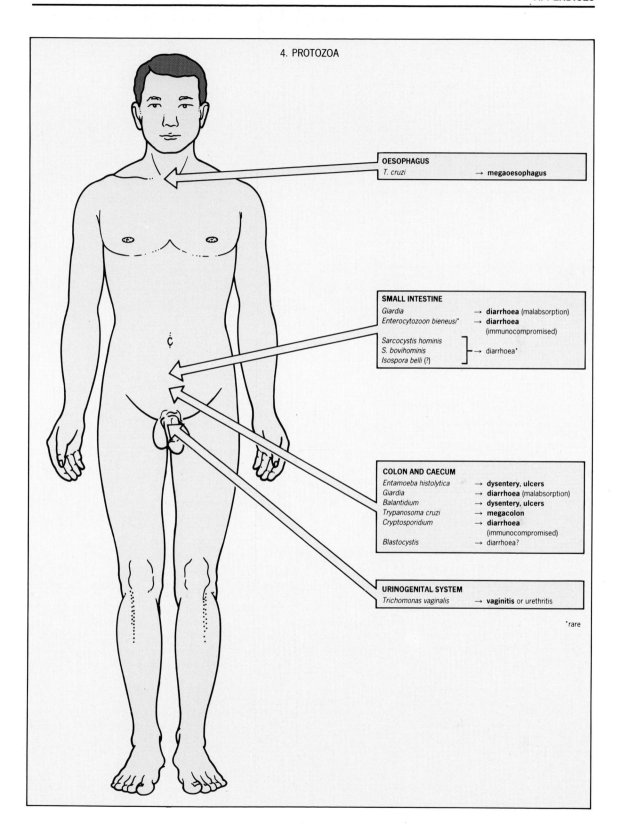

4. PROTOZOA

OESOPHAGUS
T. cruzi → **megaoesophagus**

SMALL INTESTINE
Giardia → **diarrhoea** (malabsorption)
*Enterocytozoon bieneusi** → **diarrhoea**
(immunocompromised)
Sarcocystis hominis
S. bovihominis] → diarrhoea*
Isospora belli (?)

COLON AND CAECUM
Entamoeba histolytica → **dysentery, ulcers**
Giardia → **diarrhoea** (malabsorption)
Balantidium → **dysentery, ulcers**
Trypanosoma cruzi → **megacolon**
Cryptosporidium → **diarrhoea**
(immunocompromised)
Blastocystis → diarrhoea?

URINOGENITAL SYSTEM
Trichomonas vaginalis → **vaginitis** or urethritis

*rare

5. METAZOA

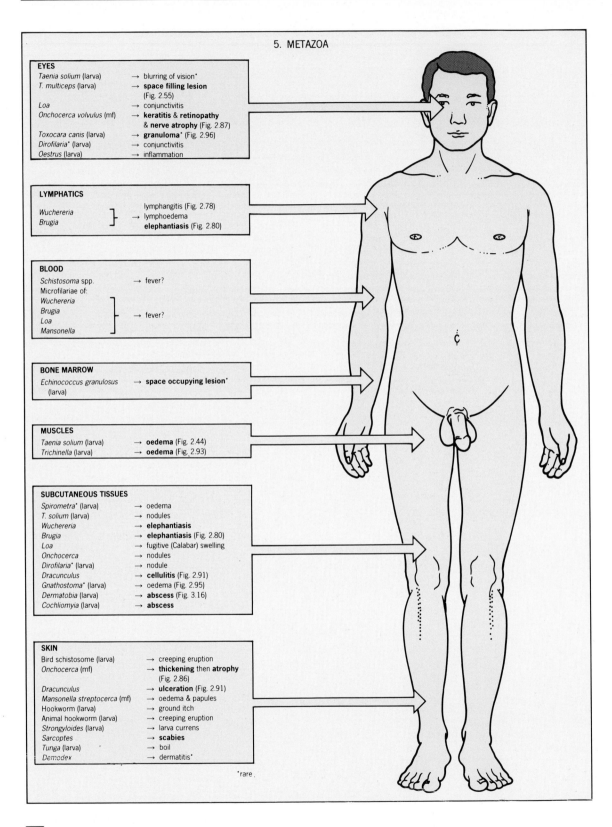

EYES

Taenia solium (larva)	→	blurring of vision*
T. multiceps (larva)	→	**space filling lesion** (Fig. 2.55)
Loa	→	conjunctivitis
Onchocerca volvulus (mf)	→	**keratitis & retinopathy & nerve atrophy** (Fig. 2.87)
Toxocara canis (larva)	→	**granuloma*** (Fig. 2.96)
*Dirofilaria** (larva)	→	conjunctivitis
Oestrus (larva)	→	inflammation

LYMPHATICS

Wuchereria
Brugia → lymphangitis (Fig. 2.78) / lymphoedema / **elephantiasis** (Fig. 2.80)

BLOOD

Schistosoma spp. → fever?
Microfilariae of:
Wuchereria
Brugia
Loa → fever?
Mansonella

BONE MARROW

Echinococcus granulosus (larva) → **space occupying lesion***

MUSCLES

Taenia solium (larva) → **oedema** (Fig. 2.44)
Trichinella (larva) → **oedema** (Fig. 2.93)

SUBCUTANEOUS TISSUES

*Spirometra** (larva)	→	oedema
T. solium (larva)	→	nodules
Wuchereria	→	**elephantiasis**
Brugia	→	**elephantiasis** (Fig. 2.80)
Loa	→	fugitive (Calabar) swelling
Onchocerca	→	nodules
*Dirofilaria** (larva)	→	nodule
Dracunculus	→	**cellulitis** (Fig. 2.91)
*Gnathostoma** (larva)	→	oedema (Fig. 2.95)
Dermatobia (larva)	→	**abscess** (Fig. 3.16)
Cochliomyia (larva)	→	**abscess**

SKIN

Bird schistosome (larva)	→	creeping eruption
Onchocerca (mf)	→	**thickening** then **atrophy** (Fig. 2.86)
Dracunculus	→	**ulceration** (Fig. 2.91)
Mansonella streptocerca (mf)	→	oedema & papules
Hookworm (larva)	→	ground itch
Animal hookworm (larva)	→	creeping eruption
Strongyloides (larva)	→	larva currens
Sarcoptes	→	**scabies**
Tunga (larva)	→	boil
Demodex	→	dermatitis*

*rare

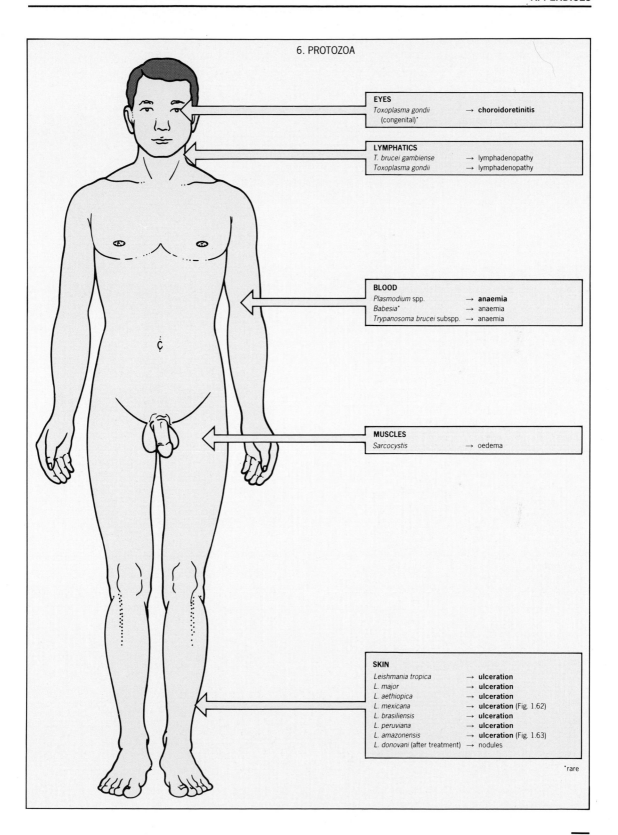

6. PROTOZOA

EYES
Toxoplasma gondii → **choroidoretinitis**
  (congenital)*

LYMPHATICS
T. brucei gambiense → lymphadenopathy
Toxoplasma gondii → lymphadenopathy

BLOOD
Plasmodium spp. → **anaemia**
*Babesia** → anaemia
Trypanosoma brucei subspp. → anaemia

MUSCLES
Sarcocystis → oedema

SKIN
Leishmania tropica → **ulceration**
L. major → **ulceration**
L. aethiopica → **ulceration**
L. mexicana → **ulceration** (Fig. 1.62)
L. brasiliensis → **ulceration**
L. peruviana → **ulceration**
L. amazonensis → **ulceration** (Fig. 1.63)
L. donovani (after treatment) → nodules

*rare

FURTHER READING
AND INDEX

FURTHER READING

General

Ash, L.R. & Orihel, T.C. (1987) *Parasites: a guide to laboratory procedures and identification*. Chicago: American Society of Clinical Pathologists/Raven Press

Ash, L.R. & Orihel, T.C. (1984) *Atlas of human parasitology*. 2nd edition. Chicago: American Society of Clinical Pathologists.

Beaver, P.C., Jung, R.C & Cupp, E.W. (1984) *Clinical Parasitology*. 9th edition. Philadelphia: Lea and Febiger.

Binford, C.H. & Connor, D.H. (1976) *Pathology of tropical and extraordinary diseases*. Vols 1 & 2. Washington: Armed Forces Institute of Pathology.

Brown, W.J. & Voge, M. (1982) *Neuropathology of Parasitic Infections*. New York: Oxford University Press.

Bryant, C. & Behm, C. (1989) *Biochemical adaptation in parasites*. London: Chapman & Hall.

Chappell, L.H. (1980) *Physiology of parasites*. Glasgow: Blackie.

Cheng, T.C. (1986) *General Parasitology*. 2nd edition. New York: Academic Press.

Cox, F.E.G. (ed) (1982) *Modern Parasitology*. Oxford: Blackwell Scientific Publications.

Despommier, D.D. & Karapelou, J.W. (1987) *Parasite life cycles*. New York: Springer-Verlag.

Englund, P.T. & Sher, A. (eds) (1988) *The Biology of Parasitism: a molecular and immunological approach*. New York: Alan Liss.

Gustafsson, L.L., Beerman, B. & Abdi, Y.A. (1987) *Handbook of drugs for tropical parasitic infections*. London: Taylor and Francis.

James, D.H. & Gilles, H.M. (1985) *Human antiparasitic drugs: pharmacology and usage*. Chichester: Wiley.

Marcial-Rojas, R.A. (ed) (1971) *Pathology of protozoal and helminthic diseases*. Baltimore: Williams and Wilkins.

Mehlhorn, H. (ed) (1988) *Parasitology in focus*. Berlin: Springer-Verlag.

Peters, W. & Gilles, H.M. (1989) *A colour atlas of tropical medicine and parasitology*. 3rd edition. London: Wolfe Medical.

Schoenfield, H. (1981) *Antiparasitic chemotherapy*. Basel: Karger.

Sturchler, D. (1988) *Endemic areas of tropical infections*. 2nd edition. Toronto: Hans Huber.

Taylor, A.E.R. & Baker, J.R. (eds) (1987) In vitro *methods for parasite cultivation*. London: Academic Press.

Urquhart, G.M. Armour, J., Duncan, J.L., Dunn, A.M. & Jennings, F.W. (1987) *Veterinary Parasitology*. Essex: Longman/New York: Churchill Livingstone.

Chapter 1

Bruce-Chwatt, L.J. (1984) *Essential Malariology*. 2nd edition. London: Heinemann Medical Books.

Gutteridge, W.E. & Coombs, G.H. (1977) *Biochemistry of Parasitic Protozoa*. London: Macmillan.

Kreier, J.P. (ed) (1977) *Parasitic Protozoa* (4 vols). New York: Academic Press.

Kreier, J.P. & Baker, J.R. (1987) *Parasitic Protozoa*. Boston: Allen & Unwin.

Molyneux, D.H. & Ashford, R.W. (1983) *The biology of* Trypanosoma *and* Leishmania, *parasites of man and domestic animals*. London: Taylor & Francis.

Peters, W & Killick-Kendrick, R. (eds) (1987) *The Leishmaniases in biology and medicine*. London: Academic Press.

Wernsdorfer, W.H. & McGregor, I. (eds) (1988) *Malaria: principles and practice of malariology.* Edinburgh: Churchill Livingstone.

Chapter 2
Arme, C & Pappas, P.W. (1983) *Biology of the Eucestoda* (2 vols). London: Academic Press.

Barrett, J. (1981) *Biochemistry of parasitic helminths.* London: Macmillan.

Crompton, D.W.T., Nesheim, M.C. & Pawlowski, Z.S. (eds) (1985) Ascaris *and its public health significance.* London: Taylor & Francis.

Flisser, A., *et. al* (eds) (1982) *Cysticercosis: present state of knowledge and perspectives.* New York: Academic Press.

Grove, D.I. (1989) *Strongyloidiasis: a major roundworm infection of man.* London: Taylor & Francis.

Jordan, P. & Webbe, G. (1982) *Schistosomiasis: epidemiology, treatment and control.* London: Heinemann Medical.

Muller, R. (1975) *Worms and disease: a manual of medical helminthology.* London: Heinemann Medical.

Rollinson, D. & Simpson, A.J.G. (1987) *The biology of schistosomes: from genes to latrines.* London: Academic Press.

Smyth, J.D. & Halton, D.W. (1983) *The physiology of trematodes.* 2nd edition. Cambridge: Cambridge University Press.

Stephenson, L.S. & Holland, C. (1987) *The impact of helminth infections on human nutrition.* London: Taylor and Francis.

Thompson, R.C.A. (ed) (1986) *The biology of* Echinococcus *and hydatid disease.* London: Allen & Unwin.

Van den Bossche, H. Thienpont, D. & Janssens, P.G. (eds) (1985) *Chemotherapy of gastrointestinal helminths.* Berlin: Springer-Verlag.

Von Bornsdorf, B. (1977) *Diphyllobothriasis in man.* London: Academic Press.

Chapter 3
Harwood, R.F. & James, M.T. (1989) *Entomology in human and animal health.* 8th edition. Pullman: Washington State University.

Kettle, D.S. (1984) *Medical and veterinary entomology.* London: Croom Helm.

Manson-Bahr, P.E.C. & Bell, D.R. (eds) (1987) Medical entomology section. In *Manson's Tropical Diseases.* 19th edition. pp. 1381-1488. London: Baillière Tindall.

Service, M. (1986) *Blood sucking insects: vectors of disease.* London: Macmillan.

Chapters 4 & 5
Desowitz, R.S. (1980) *Ova and parasites: medical parasitology for the laboratory technologist.* Hagerstown: Harper & Row.

Roitt, I, Brostoff, J. & Male, D. (1985) *Immunology.* Edinburgh: Churchill Livingstone/London: Gower Medical Publishing.

Soulsby, E.J.L. (ed) (1987) *Immune responses in parasitic infections* (4 vols). Boca Raton: CRC Press.

Walls, K. & Schantz, P. (eds) (1986) *Immunodiagnosis of parasitic diseases. I. Helminthic diseases.* New York: Academic Press.

Wakelin, D. (1984) *Immunity to Parasites: how animals control parastic infections.* London: Edward Arnold.

Wakelin, D.M. & Blackwell, J.M. (eds) (1988) *Genetics of resistance to bacterial and parasitic infection.* London: Taylor & Francis.

Warren, K.S. & Agabian, N. (eds) (1989/90) *Immunology and molecular biology of parasitic infections.* 3rd edition. Cambridge, Mass: Blackwell Scientific.